LECTURE NOTES ON DRUGS FOR DENTAL STUDENTS

LECTURE NOTES ON
DRUGS FOR DENTAL STUDENTS

TERENCE J. WILKIN

MB, ChB, MRCP
Lecturer in Therapeutics
University of Dundee, Scotland

PETER N. DAVIDSON

BDS, FDSRCSE
Lecturer in Prosthetic Dentistry
Guy's Hospital Dental School, London

With special contributions by

J. I. MURRAY LAWSON

MB, ChB, FFARCS
Consultant Anaesthetist
Ninewells Hospital and Medical School
Dundee, Scotland

D. C. HALL

MB, ChB, BChD, FDSRCSE,
FRCPath, Barrister-at-Law
Senior Lecturer, Dental Hospital
Dundee, Scotland

R. A. F. BELL

MB, ChB, DCH, MRCP
Consultant in Child Health
Horton General Hospital
Banbury, Oxon

Blackwell Scientific Publications

OXFORD LONDON EDINBURGH
MELBOURNE

© 1979 by Blackwell Scientific Publications
Osney Mead, Oxford, OX2 0EL
8 John Street, London, WC1N 2ES
9 Forest Road, Edinburgh, EH1 2QH
P.O.Box 9, North Balwyn, Victoria, Australia

First published 1979

British Library Cataloguing in Publication Data

Wilkin, Terence J
    Lecture notes on drugs for dental students.
    1. Therapeutics, Dental   2. Materia medica,
    Dental
    I. Title   II. Davidson, Peter N
    617.6'061   RK701

    ISBN 0-632-00212-3

Distributed in U.S.A. by
Blackwell Mosby Book Distributors
11830 Westline Industrial Drive
St. Louis, Missouri 63141
and in Canada by
Blackwell Mosby Book Distributors
86 Northline Road, Toronto
Ontario, M4B 3E5

Typeset by Getset Ltd., Eynsham Oxford.
Printed and bound in Great Britain by
Billing & Sons Ltd, Guildford and Worcester.

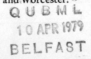

CONTENTS

Contents

PREFACE

A detailed knowledge of drugs lies in the hands of a few specialists in clinical pharmacology, while the responsibility for prescribing them rests with every dental and medical practitioner. Successful dental prescribing embodies two considerations — adequate knowledge of relevant facts and appropriate attitudes in applying them. This text book for the dental undergraduate is designed to impart basic information about both. The questions we first asked ourselves when preparing the text were, 'What facts about drugs are relevant to dentistry?'; 'What approach should be taken in presenting these facts;'; and 'What attitudes in drug prescribing are appropriate to prevailing circumstances?'.

Dentists tend to prescribe from a narrow range of drugs, notably anaesthetics (local and general), analgesics, antibiotics and topical dressings. Arguably, dental undergraduates should find little difficulty in gaining adequate knowledge of their use. However, textbooks restricted to a discussion of these drugs alone fail to take account of the fact that the dentist most frequently encounters drugs prescribed from other sources. A large proportion of his practice is liable to be taking medicines of a virtually unlimited variety. The dentist will frequently have no practical experience of the drug nor of the condition for which it was prescribed; yet in many instances the treatment he offers or the additional drugs he prescribes may have potentially serious interactions. We are therefore of the opinion that a broad familiarity with the drugs prescribed for medical conditions is mandatory for dentists.

All disease is an expression of disordered physiology and the intended action of drugs is to rectify the upset. The approach used to impart facts in this text is correspondingly physiological. Each section is disease rather than drug orientated and is prefaced by a description of the pathophysiology under consideration. Each group of drugs is then introduced in terms of the action it has on the disordered physiology. We believe that this approach will help the student develop an interest in the subject based on understanding, and aid retention of the facts by providing the rationale for the therapeutic application of drugs. In addition the content of each chapter is consolidated into a series of multiple choice questions. Most students enjoy answering MCQ's and besides providing a means of self assessment, they are fast becoming a major component of written degree examinations. Some of the questions posed (particularly those relating to attitudes rather than factual knowledge) are intended to teach, as much as to assess, so that the answer may not be explicitly stated in the text.

Preface

The optimism and euphoria over new drug developments during earlier years are now giving place to restraint and caution. The current incidence of drug-induced disease, and the realization that advances within the pharmaceutical industry have gone well beyond the capacity of the professions to master them, have led to considerable concern over present patterns of drug-prescribing. Safe prescribing is an essential element in dental care and the principles involved are stated explicitly, and often repeated, in appropriate sections of the book.

We wish to acknowledge the invaluable help of Miss Veronica Barker (Librarian, Ninewells Medical Library, Dundee), Mr P. A. C. Baigrie, Mrs Moreen Whittet and Mr. C. M. Wilkin in the preparation of this text.

INTRODUCTION

Pharmacology is a laboratory science dealing with the physical and chemical properties of drugs while thereapeutics is concerned with the application and administration of drugs in the clinical situation.

Clinical pharmacology is a relatively new science which links practical therapeutics with the observed behaviour of drugs in the living body. It has been born out of a rapidly advancing technology which allows the pharmacologist to measure *in vivo* drug concentrations, response curves, metabolism rates and patterns of excretion. Clinical pharmacology can therefore relate the known properties of a drug to a prediction of its behaviour in a particular individual, and where appropriate the text of this book refers to the more important principles involved.

Equilibria exist between the effects of the body on drugs and of drugs on the body. The points of equilibrium vary between individuals, between young and old, between male and female, healthy and infirm. Such variation accounts for the wide spectrum of drug response encountered in clinical practice. Clinical pharmacology endeavours to explain these variations and provide basic rules which can be applied by the prescriber to the clinical situation.

PART 1 · PRINCIPLES IN CLINICAL PHARMACOLOGY

1.1   THEORIES OF DRUG ACTION

CELLULAR PHYSIOLOGY AND DRUG ACTION

Living cells in the body perform two basic functions:
· The non-specific function of individual self replication by mitosis.
· The more specific biochemical activities shared by cell groups which collectively reflect the function of the organ they comprise.

Therapeutically active drugs are, by definition, substances which modify either of these cellular processes. Some drugs (e.g. cytotoxic agents) are administered for their effect on cell-division, but since most cells divide, their action tends to be general. The majority of drugs, however, are administered for their effect on specific biochemical processes by which means the function of a particular organ is enhanced (i.e. digoxin in heart failure) or reduced (e.g. carbimazole in thyrotoxicosis). Unfortunately, no drug is absolutely specific to a particular group of cells; to a varying extent all drugs modify the behaviour of cells other than those of the target organ, resulting in side-effects which may or may not be observed clinically.

In addition to modifying the function of other cells, some drugs exert their optimal therapeutic effects in dosages very close to those which will so alter the function of the target cells as to produce unwanted effects. The margin of safety between maximum efficacy and unwanted toxicity varies with different drugs and is termed the therapeutic index. Safe drugs have a high therapeutic index and toxic drugs a low index.

AGONISTS AND ANTAGONISTS

Agonists have a positive observable effect on cell function; antagonists, when used alone, generally produce no clinical effect but when used in combination with the related agonist will prevent it from acting. Narcotic analgesics are potent and valuable pain-killers. Serious respiratory depression can result from excessive dosage but is reversed within minutes of giving a specific antagonist such as naloxone.

DRUG RECEPTOR THEORY

The theory that drugs lock on to specific receptors on the surface of cell membranes has been accepted for many years, but the original proposals failed to explain all the observed facts. In particular it was not clear why nicotine first stimulates and then blocks nerve conduction or why antagonists, if they lock on to receptors which might otherwise be occupied by agonists, apparently fail to stimulate.

A more recent modification to the drug receptor theory (Paton 1960) argues that stimulation by an agonist drug results not from its presence on a receptor site but from the momentary act of combination with the receptor; once combined, no further excitation occurs. Further excitation can only occur if the drug molecule is first released from the receptor, i.e. dissociates itself.

On the assumption that the effect of a drug depends upon the number of receptor attachments it can make in unit time, the limiting factor (in the presence of unlimited drug) is necessarily the rate of dissociation. Agonists dissociate very frequently and antagonists, although usually very similar in structure to the agonists, differ from them in dissociating infrequently. Such drugs block receptors to further combinations by the agonist; their initial impact may be stimulatory (i.e. nicotine), though only feebly so, and in most cases it is not clinically observable. Further phenomena may be similarly explained. Drug action is clinically maximal at first exposure after which the effect gradually wears off, the fall off in action relating to a rising occupancy of membrane receptors. With continuing availability of the drug an equilibrium is attained between occupancy and dissociation rates. It should be clear that doubling the concentration of available drug near the critical level of total occupancy does not achieve anything like a twofold increase in the drug's effect; it may simply lead to the emergence of unwanted actions on the cells of other organs — side effects.

1.2   MECHANISMS OF DRUG TRANSFER

Whatever its presentation (e.g. tablet, mixture or injection) the active constituent of most drugs is either weak acid or weak base. Such drugs ionize to a varying extent when dissolved in water. A few drugs do not ionize at all and some are only soluble in lipids.

Physiologists speak of the major fluid compartments of the body as vascular, extracellular and intracellular. These compartments are divided off by cell boundaries, and in order to pass from one compartment to another drugs must be able to permeate these cells. In addition to the major compartments, cell boundaries also divide off the CSF from the plasma (meninges), the urine from the plasma (glomeruli and tubular epithelium), the foetal circulation from the maternal blood (placenta) and the breast milk from the plasma (acinar cells).

The ease with which a particular drug crosses these boundaries will determine its distribution within the body. For example a drug which fails entirely to cross cell boundaries will not be absorbed if swallowed and if injected intravenously will not pass beyond the vascular space.

Cell-boundaries are made of lipid material containing very fine water-filled perforations or pores. The pores of most cell membranes are too tiny to permit the passage of any but the smallest water-soluble molecules such as urea and electrolytes. The pores contained in capillary endothelial cells are, however, considerably larger and permit molecules as large as albumin to pass through by simple filtration. Since virtually all drugs are smaller than albumin, they can readily pass by simple filtration from the vascular space to the extracellular water and from the glomerular capillaries into the renal tubules. Filtration is dependent only upon the water-solubility and size of the molecule and, these conditions permitting, will occur wherever a concentration gradient exists between the two compartments.

In contrast, the blood-brain barrier, placental barrier, breast tissue and the membranes of cells (other than endothelial) dividing extracellular from intracellular compartments will not permit drugs to pass by simple filtration, but only by diffusion.

For diffusion to occur the drug must first dissolve in the cell membrane, so that this process is restricted to lipid-soluble drugs. It is the degree to which a drug is ionized that limits its lipid solubility and hence its distribution within the body. Since most drugs are weak acids or weak bases, it is clear that the environment in which the drug is placed (i.e. stomach: strongly acidic, plasma: weakly alkaline) will determine its lipid-solubility, according to the equation:

$$HD \underset{acidic}{\overset{alkaline}{\rightleftharpoons}} H^+ + D^-$$

or

$$OHD \underset{alkaline}{\overset{acidic}{\rightleftharpoons}} OH^- + D^+$$

The ease of transfer of such drugs across cell membranes is directly proportional to their concentration gradient across the cell membrane and to their lipid: water partition coefficient.

The important properties of polar (ionized) and non-polar (lipid-soluble) drugs are contrasted below.

Table 1.1 represents the extremes; in between lie the majority of drugs which exhibit varying degrees of lipid solubility and polarity.

Filtration and diffusion are passive phenomena. Occasionally drugs pass through cell boundaries by specialized active transport processes whose mechanism is selective for certain substances, requires energy and can be

Table 1.1

Property	Polar (ionized)	Non-polar (lipid-soluble)
Absorption	Poor from the gut	Well absorbed orally
Distribution	Extracellular fluid only	Total body water
Placenta)		
Blood-brain barrier)	Unable to cross	Cross easily
Breast tissue)		
Glomerular filtration	Rapid	Rapid
Tubular reabsorption	Nil	May be total
Liver metabolism	Nil	Main pathway for excretion

readily saturated. In some cases, blocking agents can be administered to antagonise the active transport of a particular substance.

1.3   THE DRUG HALF-LIFE

$t\frac{1}{2}$ is a term increasingly found in pharmaceutical literature. This section is intended to give an indication of its relevance to modern prescribing. Drug effect and toxicity are related to plasma levels. Plasma levels of many drugs can be measured directly, and the kinetics of a drug are best shown by its disappearance rate from the plasma. If the disappearance rate is slow, steady plasma levels can be achieved even by widely-spaced administration of the drug. With a drug whose elimination rate is rapid, frequent doses are necessary to maintain effective and steady plasma levels. The disappearance rate is, of course, exponential — it theoretically never disappears but simply halves in concentration every x minutes, hours or sometimes even days. The value x is known as the half-life of the drug, usually expressed as $t\frac{1}{2}$, and is obtained by injecting a bolus of the drug and taking immediate and thereafter regular measurements of its plasma concentration. A curve of concentration against time is plotted and the $t\frac{1}{2}$ obtained from the point on the graph at which the drug concentration has fallen to 50 % of the initial value.

VALUE OF MEASURING $t\frac{1}{2}$

In the marketing of a new drug, the dosage regime suggested will be based on the *mean* $t\frac{1}{2}$ established by measurement in large numbers of a random population. Such values, although useful as a guide, cannot be applied to any one individual, and the variation between individuals is often considerable.

If a drug, taken in the prescribed dosage, is found in a particular patient to be either ineffective or toxic, the clinical pharmacologist can often measure the plasma level. If this is unusually high or low, measurement of the $t\frac{1}{2}$ may provide the explanation, i.e. in the case of toxicity, the $t\frac{1}{2}$ may be unduly prolonged, pointing to unusually slow elimination as the cause. His next step is to investigate the reason.

1.4   FACTORS AFFECTING PLASMA LEVELS OF DRUGS

Drugs act at cellular level; the intensity of action depends upon their plasma concentration. Three major factors control the plasma concentration of a drug:
1. Rate of absorption.
2. Distribution within the body.
3. Rate of elimination.

Factors which influence absorption and elimination in particular are essential knowledge for the prescriber, and the important principles are outlined below. The subject is called pharmacokinetics.

ABSORPTION

Absorption deals with the transport of the drug from its site of application or administration to the bloodstream. Some drugs owe their particular usefulness to rapid absorption, others to the fact that they are not absorbed at all. Again, some drugs may be absorbed only via the parenteral route, limiting their usefulness in certain situations. (Rate and extent of absorption are two different qualities but the distinction is not often of great importance in practical therapeutics).

The factors which influence absorption are:
1. Solubility of the drug — this is partly pH dependent.
2. Concentration of drug solution used.
3. The circulation at the site of absorption. Dentists commonly use a local anaesthetic containing adrenaline. This causes local vasoconstriction, limits the anaesthetic's absorption and, preventing dispersal, retains maximal concentration at the intended site of action.
4. Absorptive surface area. The villi of the small intestine and alveoli of the lungs present enormous surface areas for the absorption of drugs given orally or by inhalation (e.g. general anaesthetics).
5. Route of administration. Intravenous injection is the most certain means of achieving maximum plasma levels of a drug in the briefest

possible time, since none of the factors which limit absorption are operative. However i.v. injection has several important disadvantages, and other routes are generally preferred.

DISTRIBUTION

Once absorbed into the bloodstream drugs are distributed and partitioned throughout the body according to their filtrability and diffusability. The plasma concentration of a drug will vary with its volume of distribution; those confined to the extracellular space achieve more than twice the concentration per dose than those distributed throughout total body water (other factors excluded). Plasma proteins (mainly albumin), fat, bone and connective tissue selectively bind many drugs and act as storage compartments, a fact of some clinical importance. Protein and tissue binding of drugs renders them inactive and the proportion bound may be as high as 98 %; this radically alters the anticipated volume of distribution and plasma concentration of active drug. Small changes in the degree of binding may result in large percentage changes in free drug concentration, and protein-bound drug complexes do not filter readily from the plasma into the interstitial fluid and renal tubular fluid (urine).

ELIMINATION

Both water-soluble (mainly polar) and lipid-soluble drugs pass readily into the glomerular filtrate. Whereas most polar substances continue on in the urine, lipid-soluble drugs are soon reabsorbed by diffusion through renal tubular cells so that very little is finally excreted. Unless a lipid-soluble drug is to remain active in the body for protracted periods of time, it must either be inactivated or rendered polar. Either or both reactions may occur, usually in the liver, by a process called drug metabolism. Drug metabolism, despite its complexity, is no more than a system of drug elimination achieved by polarizing (ionizing) the metabolites of otherwise lipid-soluble drugs.

Elimination Characteristics of
Water-soluble drugs (kidney-dependent drugs)

Drugs such as digoxin, which are water-soluble, are excreted by simple renal filtration. Factors which influence this route of excretion are:
1. Glomerular filtration rate. Renal failure will lead to accumulation unless the dosage side of the equation is proportionately reduced.
2. Affinity for plasma-proteins. Many drugs (both lipid and water-

soluble) circulate attached to plasma proteins in a dynamic equilibrium which can be expressed thus:

$$\text{Drug} + \text{Protein} \rightleftharpoons \text{DP}$$

The DP combination is too large a molecule for renal filtration. If the plasma concentration of free drug is small, and assuming that the drug is totally dependent on the kidney for excretion, the elimination rate will inevitably be slow.

3. Urinary pH. The degree of ionization of the drug will depend upon urinary pH. The elimination of phenobarbitone (and other weakly acidic drugs) can be increased by rendering the urine alkaline.

4. Tubular excretion. There are independent and *active* secretory mechanisms in the proximal renal tubules for the excretion of some acids and bases; penicillin uses this pathway in addition to simple filtration. Probenecid will block this pathway of excretion and plasma levels of penicillin can be usefully raised in the treatment of such conditions as infective endocarditis, where high concentrations of antibiotic are essential.

Elimination Characteristics of Metabolized Drugs

Since metabolism is a means of drug elimination, factors which influence its rate will affect the plasma levels of metabolized drugs accordingly. Some drugs are metabolized by specific liver enzymes; most, however, share a small number of non-specific enzymes.

Metabolism generally leads to inactivation, but some drugs such as phenacetin (mild analgesic) become pharmacologically active only after degradation. More rarely still, it is the degradation products, rather than the free drug which are toxic so that, although rapid metabolism is usually a feature of a safe drug, it may occasionally lead to toxicity.

FACTORS WHICH INFLUENCE DRUG METABOLISM

Physiological Variation

The influence of age, sex and race in themselves lead to wide variations in the rate of drug breakdown.

Interference by other drugs

The careful study of the influence of one drug on the metabolism of another has shed a great deal of light on the apparent toxicity of some drugs and the loss of effectiveness of others when used in combination.

Drugs may interact at the metabolic level in one of two ways:

Enzyme Inhibition: Many drugs share common metabolic enzymes and when present in combination compete for the limited amount of enzyme. The result depends upon the avidity of each competing drug for the enzyme system.

Enzyme Induction: Whereas some drugs competitively inhibit enzymatic breakdown, others, such as phenobarbitone in particular, stimulate enzyme production. The plasma half-life of phenobarbitone lessens with continued use (self-induction); a similar fall in $t\frac{1}{2}$ may occur with other drugs used simultaneously.

Capacity-limited metabolism

The metabolic elimination routes taken by some drugs (e.g. salicylate, phenytoin) have a limited enzyme reserve which may be exceeded in therapeutic dose, but more significantly in overdosage. The clinical effect is a dose-dependent half-life which lengthens as the dosage rises.

Genetic Factors (pharmacogenetics)

The study of pharmacogenetics has explained some anomalies of drug response encountered in clinical practice. In many cases it is a genetically determined lack of specific enzyme which accounts for the unexpected response, and unexpectedly rapid or slow rates of drug metabolism may result.

1.5   DRUG INTERACTIONS

Drug interactions may occur whenever two or more drugs are given simultaneously, and is not limited solely to effects upon metabolism. It should be remembered that not all interactions are harmful — some result in useful synergism. For instance co-trimoxazole (antibacterial agent) comprises two drugs which if used independently are bacteriostatic but in combination are bactericidal. Drug interactions may result in:

1.   Unexpected increase or decrease in drug response.
2.   Unexpectedly intense side effects.

Because many interactions go unrecognized, their true incidence is unknown. A major problem arises when a patient is discharged from hospital on drugs with inadequate information to his G.P. or dentist, either of whom may prescribe further drugs in ignorance of existing treatment, unless he takes great care to elicit the information personally.

Only a few of the important drug interactions are common but this does not belie their seriousness. The pharmacological and toxic effects of a drug are related to its free plasma concentration (i.e. concentration of unbound drug). Interaction between drugs may occur at any stage from absorption to excretion but whatever the type of interaction, the result is usually to influence plasma levels of free drug.

STAGES OF DRUG INTERACTION
(other than metabolism p.7)

Administration

Drug solutions mixed in infusion bottles may interact dangerously; e.g. calcium salts may precipitate tetracyclines, antibiotics and heparin are incompatible with hydrocortisone, dextrose reduces the effectiveness of heparin.

Drugs in the same syringe may interact — Thiopentone and suxamethonium interact chemically; if soluble insulin is placed in the same syringe as protamine zinc insulin (PZI) the excess of protamine will convert a proportion of the soluble insulin to PZI.

Absorption

The following factors may influence the passage of drugs through the gastro-intestinal mucosa.

Gut pH.
The strongly acidic gastric juice favours absorption of weak acids. By raising the stomach pH (e.g. with alkalis used in ulcer dyspepsia), the rate of absorption of such drugs as salicylates, barbiturates and warfarin will be reduced and therapeutic plasma levels may not be reached.

Chelation
Tetracyclines chelate with metals and interaction with milk (calcium), and antacids (calcium, magnesium and aluminium) may reduce their absorption; Phytic acid in certain foods can similarly bind the iron of ferrous sulphate as a phytate salt.

Note: Gastro-intestinal drug absorption is dependent on many physiological factors which can be influenced by other drugs, e.g. motility by atropine and cathartics, gut flora by antibiotics. This is a detailed study but not (at least at present) of great practical importance to therapeutics.

Tissue binding (plasma-proteins and cellular tissues)

Of primary clinical importance is the phenomenon of plasma protein binding shared by many drugs (p.6). In this context, plasma proteins can be considered as non-specific drug receptors from which there is no drug response. Drugs bind to plasma proteins with varying affinities and one can displace another.

Receptors

Drug interaction at receptors is most commonly apparent as competitive antagonism, and the dominant effect is simply a function of the relative concentrations and affinities of the interacting drugs. Many useful therapeutic agents are antagonists of naturally occurring substances, e.g. sympathetic and parasympathetic blocking agents, neuromuscular blockers.

Excretion

The factors which influence renal excretion have been discussed previously. Drugs which alter urinary pH (potassium citrate→alkaline, ammonium chloride→acid) may significantly alter the tubular reabsorption and hence ultimate excretion of a weakly ionized drug. This is only of practical significance with drugs which are excreted for the most part unchanged in the urine.

1.6   METHODS OF DRUG ADMINISTRATION

ORAL-RECTAL

Absorption via the oral mucosa (usually sublingual), stomach, small intestine, rectal mucosa (by suppository).

Advantages
Safety and convenience.

Disadvantages
Unpalatable preparations, gastric irritation, complexing with food, destruction by gastric and duodenal enzymes, breakdown by liver (the gut is drained by the portal circulation).

Sublingual absorption
Small surface area, but irritation, food complexing, enzymatic destruction

and liver breakdown are all avoided. Glyceryl Trinitrate (anti-anginal drug) is extremely effective via this route but virtually ineffective if swallowed owing to breakdown by liver.

Gastric absorption
Degree of absorption (which occurs by simple non-ionic diffusion) is strongly pH-dependent (stomach pH 1.4). Generally, drugs are better absorbed on an empty stomach. Irritant drugs, however, may be tolerated only if taken along with food.

Small Intestine
Offers a huge surface area for absorption by simple non-ionic diffusion. In an alkaline medium, basic drugs are better absorbed. The few ionized drugs which have a sufficiently small molecular size (e.g. potassium chloride, ferrous sulphate) filter readily through the intestinal wall. Some drugs which cause gastric irritation are compounded as enteric-coated preparations; the capsule is designed to pass through the stomach into the intestine before breaking up to release its contents for absorption.

Sustained-release preparations
Capsules which contain thousands of granules of the drug of widely varying size. The capsule is digested by gastric enzymes and releases the granules which dissolve at different rates with the aim of producing sustained absorption over a long period of time. The blood levels obtained from such preparations are, however, by no means predictable and may fluctuate considerably.

INJECTION

Advantages
Absorption into the bloodstream is both more rapid and more predictable than gastro-intestinal absorption. Certain drugs (e.g. Aminophylline) although well-absorbed orally may be too irritant to the stomach so that injection is the only means acceptable to the patient. Strongly-ionized drugs are not well-absorbed orally and must be given by injection. Injection is often the only practical route in patients who are unconscious, in those with gastro-intestinal disease and in emergency situations where a rapid drug response is required. Injection also avoids patient error — the lack of patient reliability in taking oral preparations is notorious, particularly in the elderly.

Disadvantages
Injection carries the danger of sepsis. Some drugs are irritant on injection (e.g. benzylpenicillin on intramuscular injection).

Safety and convenience
Generally speaking injections are less safe than oral preparations. Mistakes cannot be rectified as easily, injections are less acceptable to patients and the majority cannot be self-administered.

METHODS OF INJECTION

1. Subcutaneous
Circulation to the skin is less than that to deeper tissues and absorption slower. Insulin and adrenaline are given subcutaneously; the depot preparations of insulin are bound to large particles (e.g. protamine zinc) which further reduce the rate of absorption.

2. Intramuscular
Painful if the drug is irritant. The site must be carefully chosen to avoid vital structures (e.g. sciatic nerve in the buttock, radial nerve in the arm). Absorption can be prolonged by giving oily preparations (e.g. depot ACTH) or drugs of low solubility (e.g. procaine penicillin). The intramuscular route must be avoided in patients with a bleeding tendency (e.g. haemophilia, thrombocytopenia) owing to danger of muscle bleeding (haematoma).

3. Intravenous
An instantaneous and reliable means of achieving high blood concentrations; restricted, however, to water-soluble drugs. The intravenous route permits the use of otherwise intoleraby irritant drugs, (e.g. cytotoxic agents).

Drugs added to intravenous infusions

Experiments, particulary with antibiotics, have shown that the high blood levels obtained by intermittent intravenous injection are therapeutically more effective than the levels which result from adding the same dose of drug to a drip infusion given over similar intervals of time. In addition, many drugs interact with the infusion medium and the use of multiple constituent infusions is to be deplored.

LESS COMMONLY-USED ROUTES OF DRUG ADMINISTRATION

1. Inhalation
All maintenance general anaesthetics are given by inhalation. Many drugs,

specifically directed at lung disease, are administered by aerosol but there are inherent dangers to this (see under section on iatrogenic disease).

2. Mucous membranes
Oral, vagina, conjunctiva, rectum, Mainly used for local effect.

3. Intrathecal
Many drugs (lipid-insoluble) distribute poorly into the cerebro-spinal fluid so that direct injection at either spinal (lumbar) or brain-stem (cisternal) level is sometimes necessary, i.e. in infective meningitis and leukaemia of the meninges.

4. Topical
Many mucosal and skin disorders respond to topical applications. The commonest complication is surface sensitization to the drug. Occasionally sufficient drug is absorbed to become systemically active or toxic (e.g. topically applied corticosteroids), particularly when applied to an inflamed or ulcerated area.

PART 2 · DENTAL PRESCRIBING

2.1 THE IMPLICATIONS OF PRESCRIBING DRUGS

A drug by accepted definition, (WHO 1966) is a substance or product that is used or intended to be used to *modify* or explore *physiological systems* or pathological states *for the benefit of the patient*

MODIFY PHYSIOLOGICAL SYSTEMS

For a doctor or dentist to set about modifying physiological systems in a fellow human being is a serious undertaking, yet the public demand for medication in the form of drugs (and the profession's willingness to prescribe them!) suggests that the implications are not always fully grasped. Safe prescribing is an essential part of good patient care and prescribing in ignorance amounts to negligence. Many of the generalizations which can be made in relation to drug prescribing are, in reality, little more than commonsense:

1 It is better practice to withhold drugs entirely than to create illness through their use.

2 The vast numbers of individual drugs marketed in fact derive from a much smaller number of drug groups. Within each group, member drugs often differ little and it is far safer to gain knowlege and experience with a single representative of the group than attempt to be master of them all.

3 When in search of prescribing information, use a standard pharmacopoeia (e.g. Dental Practitioner's Formulary, Martindale's Pharmacopoeia). While manufacturers' literature is usually the truth, it is not always the whole truth.

4 Commercial pressures are strong. New drugs must be assessed critically by the prescriber. Quotations from the journals made by manufacturers may be convincing but are sometimes lacking in context. It is worth knowing something of the principles of good design in clinical trials; more important perhaps is to ensure that the journals quoted in advertising literature are reputable and well known.

There is no room for complacency in a situation where medicine is contributing to the incidence of disease and the prescriber must never be in doubt about the properties of a drug he intends to prescribe.

BENEFIT TO THE PATIENT

The drug prescriber bears a unique responsibility in deciding on the appropriate treatment of disease. Given a sound understanding of pharmacological principles he is in a position to rationalize his approach. Simple ailments in general require simple measures and where drugs are indicated, simple drugs. Advantage to the patient can only result where the side-effects of a drug are outweighed by the cure of disease or relief of symptoms. Side-effects must involve long as well as short term considerations. Whatever the situation, the prescriber must be certain in his own mind that the patient will benefit from his prescriptions; the incidence of predictable iatrogenic disease suggests that many are not. Perhaps the most important distinction between good and bad prescribing is the ability to withold drugs where there is no firm indication for their use.

PRINCIPLES OF PRESCRIBING

If the following 'rules of thumb' are strictly adhered to, the incidence of drug-induced disease (euphemistically called 'therapeutic misadventures') should be reduced to a minimum.

1   Do not prescribe a drug, the metabolism and route of excretion of which you are ignorant.

2   Use the lowest effective dose (owing to the increased and often unpredictable sensitivity to drugs in old age, standard dosages quoted may be misleading).

3   Ensure that the benefits expected of the drug are likely to outweigh its side-effects.

4   Continually review the clinical indications for the drug rather than issue repeat prescriptions.

5   Use a minimum number of drugs at any one time.

2.2   IATROGENIC DISEASE

Disease or discomfort caused by the dentist could take many forms but one of mounting importance in medicine generally is that due to the misuse of drugs. Drug-induced (iatrogenic) disease may result from insufficient knowledge on the part of the prescriber, misunderstanding by the patient of the dosage to be taken, aberrations on the part of the patient or from unexpected (idiosyncratic) response. Commonly failure of communication between physician and dentist is at the root of the problem.

INCIDENCE OF IATROGENIC REACTIONS

Accuracy in assessment of incidence depends on the quality of information obtainable. The Medicines Commission makes available to practitioners
yellow cards on which abnormal reactions to drugs may be noted and filed
at a central office (Fig. 2.1). Such a system is inevitably underused and in
any event tends to focus on unexpected reactions, leaving undocumented
the therapeutic accidents which occur through negligence or misuse. Most
of the information available centres on medical rather than dental prescribing but the lessons learnt from medical experience can equally well be
applied to help the dentist.

Studies show that drug-induced disease is commonly due only to a
small number of constant offenders (anticoagulants, corticosteroids,
phenlybutazone and phenacetin) and that polypharmacy is a high-risk
factor. Also important are age (the elderly are more susceptible to adverse
reactions), and concomitant disease.

A number of factors liable in practice to lead to drug-induced disease
can be identified, in both the patient and the prescribing practitioner.

The Patient

While it is important to identify the types of drug most likely to cause
complication, and to avoid them if at all possible, it is equally necessary to
identify and evaluate the poor-risk patient who is liable to administer
incorrectly the drugs he has been prescribed. Perpetual drug abusers are
often well known to their doctors; less obvious problem groups are those
with failing eyesight (who may not admit the fact), the elderly who may
easily become confused by all but the simplest drug regimens, those of low
intelligence, the unreliable (a characteristic which may be reflected to
some extent in their failure to attend for appointments), those with
psychiatric disorders, and children.

Fortunately (from the toxicity viewpoint) many of the above situations
lead to failure to take the drug rather than to overdosage.

The Practitioner

(a) *Unfamiliarity*
There is clearly a major problem set by the variety and sophistication of
drugs currently offered by the pharmaceutical industry. No practitioner
can be expected to remember the characteristics of them all and dentists
may be tempted to prescribe drugs about which they in fact know very
little. Since virtually no drug is without side-effects, drug-induced disease
is from time to time an inevitable result. The answer clearly is to be

selective, to resist the pressures of the pharmaceutical industry and to prescribe from a small number of proven preparations with which the prescriber has gained familiarity through repeated experience (one reason for the Dental Formulary).

(b) *Polypharmacy*

Surveys suggest that hospitalized patients receive on average five drugs simultaneously, and 10 % are taking no less than ten drugs at any one time! In a medicine-dependent society the pressures on family practitioners to treat all symptoms with drugs is likewise considerable, and multiple symptomatology often leads to multiple drug therapy. The potential for drug interaction with resulting toxicity is clear but an even greater problem exists where a failure in communication between two practitioners (e.g. doctor and dentist) permits one to prescribe in ignorance of the drugs the other has administered.

In practice, despite the theoretical risks involved, illness through drug *interaction* accounts for only a small part of the problem caused by iatrogenic disease. Examples of drug-induced disease relevant to dental practice are listed on p.20. Of particular importance for the dentist to recognize are aplastic anaemia, agranulocytosis, drug-induced disorders of clotting and jaundice.

2.3 THE INDIVIDUALIZATION OF DRUG THERAPY

If drugs always elicited the responses expected of them, the practitioner's job would be much easier and his responsibilities as a prescriber considerably lighter. The fact is, however, that drugs commonly produce either no response at all or an intensity or type of response far different from that anticipated.

Much of the difficulty stems from the traditional concepts of dosage regimes. While guide-lines as to the dose for a particular drug are clearly essential, many sources of reference are dogmatic; they often fail to emphasize the wide variation between individuals in their response to a standard dosage of a particular drug, and the consequent need for flexibility. Many drugs are discarded by prescribers because they 'don't work.' The more likely explanation is that optimum dosage is not achieved because the dose 'given in the book' is too strictly adhered to.

With the advent of drug plasma level measurements came the first objective evidence of how wide individual variation can be. Physicians are used to manipulating dosage according to individual response for certain groups of drugs (e.g. antihypertensive drugs, corticosteroids, anti-thyroid

IN CONFIDENCE —REPORT ON SUSPECTED ADVERSE DRUG REACTIONS

1. Please report all reactions to recently introduced drugs and serious or unusual reactions to other drugs. (Vaccines should be regarded as drugs.)
2. Record on the top line the drug you suspect of causing the adverse reaction.
3. Record all other drugs, including self—medication, taken in the previous 3 months. With congenital abnormalities, record all drugs taken during pregnancy.
4. Do not be deterred from reporting because some details are not known.

NAME OF PATIENT (To allow linkage with other reports for same patient. Also give record number for hospital patient)				SEX	AGE OR DATE OF BIRTH	WEIGHT
DRUGS * (Give brand name if known)	ROUTE	DAILY DOSE	DATE STARTED	DATE ENDED	INDICATIONS	
*For Vaccines give Batch No.						

REACTIONS	STARTED	ENDED	OUTCOME (e.g. fatal, recovered)

ADDITIONAL NOTES

REPORTING DOCTOR

Name ————

Address ————

Tel No. ————

Signature ————

Date ————

Fig. 2.1 The reply paid card available from the Medical Assessor of the Committee on Safety of Medicines for the purpose of reporting adverse reactions to drugs observed in medical or dental patients.

drugs) but in order to achieve optimum response it is probably necessary to do so in most therapeutic situations.

FACTORS INFLUENCING DRUG RESPONSE

Several factors can be identified which may explain the failure of a drug to achieve its anticipated response. Completely inappropriate dosage is of course one of them; others include:

Non-compliance
This is the commonest. For a variety of reasons, social, personal and environmental, patients may fail to take a drug as prescribed. Forgetfulness, and failure to realize the significance of the drug's action are frequent causes.

Age (see also p.26)
The ageing process is one of physiological change and the response to drugs in the elderly frequently alters accordingly. Side effects are often more intense and appear at lower dosages. Forgetfulness or confusion, particulary if several drugs are being prescribed simultaneously, may compound the problem. Infants and children also respond differently to drugs than the adult.

Idiosyncracy
Such reactions, mostly allergic and sometimes serious, are by their nature unavoidable in the first instance. It is the responsibility of the prescriber to document the offending drug in such a way that the patient never receives it again. This implies a means of communication between dentist and doctor; if a dentist notes allergy in a child to the penicillin he has prescribed, he must ensure:
a.   That both the child and his parents know that penicillin must never again be prescribed.
b.   That the child's G.P. has notification of the fact *by letter*.

Drug-disease interactions
Throughout this book are cited situations in which the use of certain drugs is contra-indicated. In many instances the contra-indications are disease states in which it is known that the drug is liable to have unpleasant or toxic effects. Clearly a knowledge of these interactions and an understanding of the toxicology are important in the interests of safe prescribing.

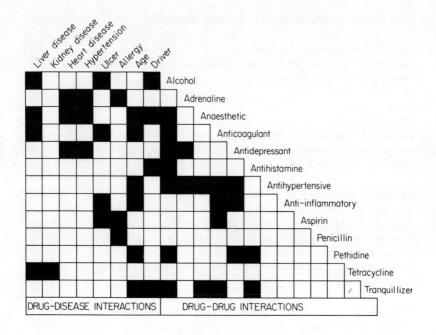

Table 2.1 Common drug-drug and drug-disease interactions.

2.4 PRESCRIBING FOR CHILDREN
BY R. A. F. BELL

The dental surgeon spends a large part of his working life treating children, and he will prescribe drugs for some of them. In addition some of his patients will be receiving treatment from their family doctors, which may itself alter reactions to dental disease or to its treatment. The dentist should therefore have some knowledge of the special problems of drug therapy in childhood.

RETICULOSES (p.182)

Children suffering from acute lymphoblastic leukaemia, who, only a generation ago, would have died within a few weeks, now usually survive for years and some are cured completely. Treatment involves the use of toxic drugs such as steroids and antimetabolites in high dosage over long periods, and the child may suffer incapacitating side-effects.

Most of these drugs, as well as the disease itself, predispose the patient to infections, often due to organisms which are relatively innocuous to healthy people. This reduced ability to resist infection makes a high standard of dental care most desirable, and the dental surgeon caring for such children can contribute much to the child's health. Recognition of leukaemia as a cause of swollen gums or an ulcerated throat may enable the condition to be treated earlier than might otherwise have happened; similarly the dentist's recognition of methotrexate-induced oral ulceration may enable the dosage to be modified and the child's condition to improve, or the ulceration to be relieved by the use of folinic acid mouthwashes. Other conditions such as drug-induced candidiasis may also be recognized and treated.

Many of the drugs used in treating leukaemia cause thrombocytopenia, so extractions are usually performed in hospital, as platelet transfusions may be required.

EPILEPSY (p.186)

If the child is forbidden to take anything by mouth on the morning he is to receive a general anaesthetic he will not receive his morning dose of anticonvulsants. As he tends to go to bed earlier than his parents, this can mean that a period of 16hr may have elapsed since he last received his medicine, with the consequent risk of a convulsion.

DOSAGE CONSIDERATIONS

While the infant has immature metabolic and excretory mechanisms for dealing with many drugs, the child of toddler age and upwards has systems for disposing of drugs which are similar to those of adults, assuming that due allowance is made for the child's size. There are exceptions, such as digoxin and the phenothiazines, in which the child's tissues themselves have different sensitivities to the drugs from those of adults.

Most drugs are initially distributed throughout the extracellular fluid, (p.2) and as this compartment is relatively larger in childhood than in the adult, calculations of dosage are better related to the two-thirds power of body weight than to the weight itself. As it happens, the body surface area bears this same relationship to body weight and the student will encounter many references advocating this means of calculating dosage. However laudable that may be, a nomogram for calculating body surface area is not always available and it is suggested that the proportion chart in Table 2.2 should be used.

Table 2.2

Age	Percent of adult dose
1 year	25
3 years	33
7 years	50
10 years	60
14 years and over	100

There are many other ways of calculating drug dosage, and no single one is appropriate to every circumstance; whatever method is used, it is essential that the dose be checked with a reliable source of information, such as the *Dental Practitioners' Formulary* or the manufacturer's literature.

Despite such calculations, it is still possible that the child will receive an incorrect dose, due to problems of children themselves: children are liable to vomit, especially after oral medicines, and therefore if reliable results are to be obtained, the drug must often by given by injection. Similarly the actual administration of medicines may be vigorously resisted, with dispersal of the drug beyond the sites intended. Alternatively, a child may swallow the entire prescribed course of treatment while left unattended.

2.5   PRESCRIBING IN PREGNANCY
BY R. A. F. BELL

As it is considered desirable that expectant mothers should enjoy the highest possible standards of health, their dental care is made freely available and the dental surgeon is frequently liable to encounter pregnant women in his practice. It is therefore necessary that he should have some knowledge of the special problems involved in the care of such patients, and particularly so with regard to the use of drugs.

The risks engendered by the administration of medicines to pregnant women were tragically highlighted by the thalidomide disaster of the late 1950's and early 1960's. Thalidomide was a hypnotic-sedative drug which seemed to be so safe that, no matter how high the dose, it would not seriously harm the patient. In view of this it seemed the ideal hypnotic and was extensively advertised and prescribed throughout the world, except interestingly enough, the USA, where its tendency to produce a peripheral neuropathy had led to its rejection by the Food and Drugs Administration. It was not until the epidemic of children born with gross limb malformations — phocomelia — and other abnormalities such as ear defects, intestinal atresias and heart defects, was studied that the link with thalidomide was made.

It is quite clear that the decision to prescribe a drug (especially if newly introduced) to pregnant women must be made only after weighing carefully the special risks in pregnancy against the distress of withholding it; seen in this light the prescription of a sedative drug to a pregnant woman to alleviate mild symptoms of irritability must seem distinctly undesirable.

Not every expectant mother has reached the stage where she realizes she is pregnant. Furthermore she may not admit pregnancy, especially if she is either single or widowed. It is therefore probably wise to consider any woman from the age of thirteen to fifty to be potentially pregnant and to restrict one's prescribing accordingly.

Drugs given to the mother reach the foetus selectively by crossing the placenta, just like the many substances that provide for its nutrition; for many years the term placental barrier has been used but the term barrier has given undeserved reassurance. Highly-ionized substances cross with difficulty while lipid soluble ones cross readily. However, early in pregnancy, when the embryonic cells are dividing rapidly, even low concentrations of certain teratogenic substances may have devastating effects; so even drugs which cross the placenta poorly may cause harm.

A drug given early in pregnancy may affect the foetus in several ways:
· It may be so damaging that the embryo is aborted (it would then be an

aborting agent),
· It may produce some gross anatomical defect, or
· It may cause a more subtle defect which is less easily detected (covert embryopathy).
· It may have no effect at all.
    The degree of damage may be partly related to dosage.

SPECIFIC DRUGS

CORTICOSTEROIDS (Cortisone, Cortisol, Prednisolone Betamethasone, p.156)

When these drugs are used in the usual dosage, there appears to be little risk of congenital malformation, apart from a possible slightly increased incidence of cleft palate.

ANTIMICROBIAL DRUGS

These drugs are used to destroy, or inhibit the division of microbial cells, and the possibility of such drugs having similar effects on the rapidly-growing cells of an embryo is evident. Fortunately, such happenings rarely occur in human subjects, although they have been demonstrated in certain animals.

Co-trimoxazole (p.123)

Both of the constituents (sulphamethoxazole and trimethoprim) interfere with folic acid synthesis in the bacterial cell. Deficiency of folic acid may predispose to teratogenicity in the foetus and high doses of trimethoprim have been shown to produce congenital abnormalities in rats. While no such abnormalities in humans have been attributed to co-trimoxazole, it would seem reasonable to avoid giving this drug combination at present to pregnant women, unless there is no safer alternative.

Sulphonamides (p.123)

The long-acting sulphonamides are highly protein bound; while this to some extent prevents their crossing the placenta, they may, if given near term, compete with bilirubin for binding sites on serum albumin. This can predispose the infant to kernicterus, a severe neurological condition caused by unconjugated bilirubin being deposited in the infant's brain.

Aminoglycosides

(Streptomycin, Neomycin, Kanamycin and Gentamycin [p.121]): are nephrotoxic and neurotoxic, and infants have been born with eighth cranial nerve damage after treatment of the mother with streptomycin during pregnancy.

Penicillins (p.113) and Cephalosporins (p.118)

These antibiotics seem very safe in pregnancy unless, of course, the mother is allergic to them.

Tetracyclines (p.122)

The deleterious effect of tetracyclines on the teeth of growing children is well known. As the teeth are forming in utero, and tetracyclines cross the placenta, these effects may occur when a pregnant woman is given tetracycline during the period of tooth crown formation, from the fourth month of gestation onwards. The result is discolouration of the teeth.

Tetracyclines have also been implicated as a cause of congenital cataract. Maternal deaths have, rarely, followed its use. Tetracyclines should only be prescribed during pregnancy if there is no alternative.

Erythromycin

The use of this drug in pregnancy has been associated with abnormal liver function tests in the infants, but such effects have not been ascribed to any other members of the erythromycin group.

Metronidazole

First introduced for Trichomonas vaginalis infections and effective in the treatment of acute ulcerative gingivitis (Vincent's Angina). It would appear to be quite safe to the foetus, although it is recommended that the shortest possible course be used. The patient should be advised to avoid alcohol during the course of treatment as mild disulfiram-like reactions may occur (Disulfiram or 'Antabuse' has been used in alcoholism because of the very disagreeable response that results from the combination).

ANALGESICS

Salicylates (p.152)

Although aspirin is taken frequently without untoward effects, the salicylate group of drugs may not be as safe as previously considered. There have been reports of congenital malformations of the alimentary tract, central nervous system and limbs following their use, and when taken later in pregnancy, salicylates can predispose to bleeding in the foetus by interfering with platelet aggregation and factor XII formation. Salicylates, like the long-acting sulphonamides, may compete for bilirubin binding sites on plasma proteins.

HYPNOTICS, SEDATIVES AND ANTICONVULSANTS

The very nature of the conditions for which these drugs are prescribed means that they are taken over long periods of time, often before the patient knows she is pregnant. Both phenytoin and phenobarbitone given during pregnancy produce a small but definite increase in congenital abnormalities such as cleft lip and palate and the incidence is greater when phenobarbitone and phenytoin are given in combination. However, the chance of congenital defect may be outweighed by the risk to the foetus from a maternal convulsion following withdrawal of anticonvulsants.

ANAESTHETICS

Although general anaesthetics cross the placenta readily, they do not usually harm the infant, unless the procedure is associated with shock or anoxia, when the reduction of placental blood flow may cause damage to the foetus, especially to its brain. However, theatre nurses and anaesthetists, who are exposed to halothane in the course of their work, have an increased incidence of spontaneous abortion and foetal abnormality.

2.6   PRESCRIBING FOR THE ELDERLY

Drug adverse reactions and frank iatrogenic disease are more frequent in the elderly population. A number of factors may be responsible:
1   The percentage of elderly patients in the population is increasing.
2   In contrast to the acute diseases of youth, the diseases of old age are usually chronic and frequently multiple.
3   The quantity of drugs prescribed to the elderly is rising and the combinations are becoming increasingly varied. Although the elderly represent

only 12 % of the population, they account for 30 % of NHS drug expenditure.

4 The elderly are more susceptible to the adverse reactions of drugs and metabolize them differently.

5 ' Forgetfulness and confusion (which may in themselves be drug-mediated) may lead to incorrect drug identification by the patient or excessive dosage. Non-compliance (failure to take the drug as prescribed) remains the commonest cause of therapeutic failure in all age groups.

The dentist is less likely than the physician to serve a large geriatric practice but he must still take the utmost care when prescribing.

2.7   THE DENTAL PRACTITIONERS' FORMULARY AND THE LAWS RELATING TO DRUGS AND THEIR PRESCRIPTION BY D. C. HALL

THE BRITISH NATIONAL FORMULARY

In 1946 the Joint Formulary Committee was set up to simplify prescribing. It became inevitable after the advent of the National Health Service in 1948 that a Formulary for dentists was needed, 'for use in the National Health Service'. The Dental Practitioners Formulary (DPF) is issued free to all dentists practicing under the Health Service.

TERMS OF SERVICE

By placing his name on a 'Dental List' under the National Health Service a dentist undertakes to comply with the 'Terms of Service' made under the Act, which require that:

1 A practitioner has the duty to prescribe, on a form (F.P.14 in England and Wales, E.C.14 in Scotland) provided by the Area Health Authority, any drug necessary during the course of treatment from a list of approved drugs. The prescription has to be signed by the practitioner or his deputy or assistant and must not be written so as to direct the chemist to refer to a previous order.

2 If a deputy or assistant signs he must add the name of the practitioner for whom he acts.

3 A National Health Service form must only be used for a patient who is under treatment within the Service.

Once this duty is recognized, the dentist need not consider, and in fact cannot prescribe, any drug under the National Health Service other than those in the DPF. If he considers another drug would be helpful, he can prescribe it privately or ask the patient's doctor to issue an NHS prescription, as the doctor is not so restricted in his prescribing.

Where the dentist has omitted to indicate the strength or quantity of the preparation to be dispensed, the Pharmacist will attempt to contact him and have him initial the change later. Where this is not possible the Pharmacist will use his own professional judgement. These arrangements are designed to expedite dispensing. It has also been agreed that the F.P.14 and E.C.14 prescription sheets will contain a box to indicate the number of days treatment the prescription is intended to cover. This is in conformity with medical prescriptions but its use is optional.

Dentists no less than doctors are bound by the various laws regulating drugs. The right to prescribe and administer drugs to his patients is conferred on a dentist by his registration with the General Dental Council. This right carries obligations and apart from the legal consequences, abuse of the responsibility can lead to the erasure of his name from the Dental Register.

In recent years the worsening problems of drug abuse and addiction have been the subject of considerable concern both to the health professions and the Home Office. One aspect is the ready availability of addictive and psychotropic drugs to the public and between 1968 and 1972 three new Acts, designed to replace the previous law on the subject, received the Royal Assent. These Acts are:

1   The Medicines Act of 1968
2   The Misuse of Drugs Act of 1971
3   The Poisons Act of 1972

Although dentists prescribe little by comparison with doctors, these Acts remain relevant and will be considered in some detail.

THE MEDICINES ACT OF 1968

This Act has only oblique application to dentistry but is of such importance to pharmaceutical practice that its substance should be known to dentists. Its purpose is to regulate the manufacture, distribution, importation, exportation and promotion of human medicines, veterinary medicines and medicated foodstuffs for animals. In essence it demands that a licence be granted before a new drug can be promoted or even researched. The Act defines the terms for such a licence.

The UK Ministers of Health and Agriculture & Fisheries are responsible for administering the Act but they have the benefit of advice from the Medicines Commission set up under the Act.

Terms of the Act

A Medicinal Product (not medicine) is any substance or article — not being an instrument, apparatus or appliance — which is manufactured, sold, supplied, imported or exported for use wholly or mainly in either or both the following ways:

· By being administered to one or more human beings or animals for a medicinal purpose.

· As an ingredient in an article or substance for such administration, when the ingredient is used in a pharmacy or a hospital, or in a business where herbal remedies are sold by retail or by a practitioner, that is a doctor, dentist or veterinary surgeon.

The Medicines Commission

A body corporate appointed by the Ministers to advise them on the administration of the Act and on any matters relating to medicinal products.

It comprises at least eight members, one or more from each of the following professions:
(a) Medicine; (b) Veterinary Science; (c) Pharmacy; (d) Chemistry and (e) Pharmaceutical Industry.

The primary concern of the Commission is with safety rather than efficacy of drugs. All dentists should be aware of the arrangements in force for the recording of adverse reaction to drugs (p.18). The Commission is also required to make recommendations regarding the preparation of future edition of the *British Pharmacopoeia.*

Enforcement

Primary enforcement rests with the Ministers; but they may delegate powers, e.g. to Pharmaceutical Society.

Right of Entry and Legal Proceedings

An enforcement officer is given wide powers to ensure that the Act is being observed and has a right of entry into appropriate premises. Any legal proceedings by the Ministers must be taken within 12 months of receiving information.

The Licencing System

Part II of the Act sets out the licencing requirements. Without the appropriate licence it is not lawful for any person to sell, supply, export, import or manufacture any medicinal product. This Act marks a radical change in attitude. Prior to it anyone could market, manufacture, sell or promote any drug and its use was only restricted when it was found to be harmful and/or undesirable; by which time it could have done untold harm.

While a detailed knowledge of the regulations is not necessary, an understanding in broad outline is advisable. The following licences are required:

1   A Product Licence to:
    (a) import or export
    (b) sell or supply
    (c) to compound.
2   Manufacture Licence to manufacture or assemble a product.
3   Wholesale Dealer's Licence for wholesale transactions.
4   Clinical Trial and Animal Test Certificate: required to conduct animal or human trials of a drug.

· Transitional Arrangements: made to cover substances already on the market or in the process of being developed when the Act came into force.

· Exemptions: provided so as not to hamper unduly doctors, dentists or other interested parties.

· Sales Promotion: under the Act the Minister is given wide powers to prevent misleading claims, and to ensure adequate information about medicinal products by (1) advertisements, and (2) representations.

· Data Sheets: whenever a commercially-interested party advertises to practitioners, it must also offer a data sheet. The representative must not visit the practitioner to promote his product unless a data sheet has been sent. The contents of the data sheet are prescribed by the Act and must be complied with.

· Dealing with Medicinal Products: retail dealings are generally permitted only through Registered Pharmacists. Certain items however are exempt; Hospitals, Clinics, Nurses, Midwives and Dispensing Practitioners may dispense certain drugs.

· Herbal Remedies: also receive special treatment.

· 'Prescription Only' Products: Certain medicinal products may only be supplied on prescription. Prescribing restrictions do not apply to Dentists or Doctors supplying these products personally to the patient.

2.7.4   THE MISUSE OF DRUGS ACT 1971

This Act sets up an Advisory Council to advise the Minister (Secretary of State for Home Department). The Council comprises 20 members from Medicine, Dentistry, Veterinary Science, Pharmacy, Chemistry and persons with wide experience in social problems of drug dependency. They have to keep under review drugs that are, or are likely to be misused and cause harm, physical or social, and advise the Minister accordingly. Controlled Drugs are listed in Schedule II of the Act. They are divided into three classes, A, B and C, in decreasing degrees of harmfulness, but this division is solely for the purpose of determining penalties under the Act. Their transportation and exportation is limited by licence.

Production, supplying, possession and cultivation of cannabis (hemp) is illegal unless authorized by the Secretary of State.

The Act authorizes the Minister to call upon anyone with lawful possession to supply information as to drugs administered, supplied or prescribed.

Irresponsible Prescribing

If the Secretary of State is of the opinion that a practitioner has been guilty of acting in an irresponsible manner, he may make an order prohibiting him dealing in all, or certain Controlled Drugs. The Secretary of State has a Professional Panel to advise him on this matter. Such orders are published in the *London Gazette* (also Edinburgh, Belfast). Schedule 4 of the Act gives a tabulated summary of the offences under the Act and the penalties applicable to them according to whether the drug involved is in Class A, B or C.

Powers of the Secretary of State

He has powers to make regulations by Statutory Instruments; to grant licences under the Act and to make provisions under the Customs and Excise Act 1952 regarding importation and exportation: in short to prevent unlawful and permit lawful use of Controlled Drugs.

Schedules to the Regulations

The Act and regulations made under it became effective in 1973. There are five schedules to the regulations (1973); these must not be confused with the schedules of the Act itself. Nos I-IV divide the drugs controlled by the Act into four schedules each subject to different requirements, while No. V enacts the forms of the Registers to be maintained for obtaining and supplying controlled drugs.

Schedule I: This contains certain popular remedies not intended for injection which contain small amounts of drugs which in bulk are subject to more stringent controls. No records are required and no rules as to safe custody apply. They are available on Prescription only.

Schedule II: This contains a list of over 100 drugs and includes cocaine, heroin, opium, methadone, morphine, pethidine and the amphetamines. (For rules relating to prescribing Schedule II drugs, see p.32).

Schedule III: Not relevant to dentistry.

Schedule IV: This lists substances subject to the most rigorous control such as cannabis and the hallucinogens. The use of any drug in this schedule requires a special licence and the dentist is very unlikely to prescribe them.

Schedule V: An entry in a register of Controlled Drugs must be made in respect of any quantity of a Schedule II and IV drug (Tables 2.3 and 2.4). A separate register must be maintained in respect of each class of drug. These books are open to inspection by a legally authorized inspector. They must be preserved for 2 years after the last entry.

Table 2.3 Entries to be made in case of obtaining Controlled Drugs

Date on which supply was received	Name/Address of person or firm from whom obtained	Amount obtained	Form in which obtained

Table 2.4 Entries to be made in case of supplying Controlled Drugs

Date on which transaction was effected	Name/Address of person or firm from whom supplied	Particulars as to licence or authority of person or firm supplied to be in possession	Amount supplied	Form in which supplied

RULES FOR PRESCRIBING SCHEDULE II DRUGS BY A DENTIST

THE PRESCRIPTION

· Must be in ink or other indelible substance (Biro) and signed and dated by the dentist personally.

· Name and address of person to whom the drug is to be given, in dentists own writing.

· Name and address of prescribing dentist unless appropriate National Health Service prescription form is used.

· Be endorsed 'For dental treatment only'.

· The dose and when to be taken, as well as the strength of pills, capsules, etc. and the total quantity and/or total number of unit dosages in figures and words (as in a cheque) of the controlled drug to be supplied, in the dentists own handwriting.

· When a total quantity is to be dispensed by instalments, the directions as to amounts and intervals between instalments and the total of all the instalments must be given.

N.B. Normally a National Health Service prescription may not be dispensed by instalments.

THE POISONS ACT OF 1972

This Act covers the sale and possession of non-medicinal poisons. The Act does not unduly affect a Dentist in the practice of his profession, but will of course apply to him in relation to his private use of poisons for his garden and other purposes.

PRINCIPLES IN WRITING A PRESCRIPTION

It is necessary to convey to the dispensing pharmacist:
· The identification of the patient, and age if under twelve years.
· The name of the preparation, its strength and the quantity to be dispensed.
· The number of times per day and route by which it is to be taken, and whether before or after meals.
· The name of the prescribing dentist.
· The date.
   Ideally the prescription should all be printed; many would consider printing of the drug name mandatory.

SPECIMEN PRIVATE PRESCRIPTION (SCHEDULED DRUG)

```
                                          J. Entwistle B.D.S.,
                                                6 Undergate
                                                     Dundee

                                          28th February 1978

Mrs. H. Brown
4 Fountainbrae
Monifieth

R           Send 12 Tabs PETHIDINE B.P. 25mg
 x          Take 2 tabs at night
            'For dental treatment only'
            Total amount pethidine 300mg

                                          J. Entwistle B.D.S.
```

Note
The approved (or proper) name of a preparation should appear on prescription forms and will apply unless the practitioner deletes it.

SPECIMEN PRESCRIPTION (NON-SCHEDULED DRUG)

J. Smith
4 Side Street
Downfield

R   Tabs PHENOXYMETHYLPENICILLIN 250 mg
x   Send 20
               Take 1 tab qid before meals

A. Jones B.D.S.
28 February 1978

COMMONLY-USED ABBREVIATIONS

a.c	(ante cibum), before meals
b.d. or b.i.d.	(bis in die), twice daily
BNF	British National Formulary
BP	British Pharmacopoeia
B.P.C.	British Pharmaceutical Codex
D.P.F.	Dental Practitioners' Formulary
I.M.	Intramuscularly
I.U.	International Unit
I.V.	Intravenously
mitte	Send
N.P.	(Nomen proprium) Proper name
p.c.	(post cibum), after meals
p.r.n.	(pro re nata) as required
q.d.s or q.i.d.	(quattuor in die) four times daily
R$_x$	(Recipe) Take thou
S.C.	Subcutaneously
Sig	(Sigillum) let it be written
Stat.	Immediately
t.d.s. or t.i.d.	(ter in die), thrice daily

PART 3 · DENTAL ANAESTHESIA

3.1 MODE OF ACTION OF GENERAL ANAESTHETICS
BY J. I. MURRAY LAWSON

The purpose of this section is to impart a basic knowledge of the drugs used for general anaesthesia and sedation in the dental outpatient and of the principles of the techniques employed. It cannot be emphasized too strongly that, although many general anaesthetics are still administered by general dental (and medical) practitioners with no special training in the subject, this is properly a field for the specialist anaesthetist. He alone possesses a full appreciation of the potential clinical effect of anaesthetic agents and the constantly-practised ability to manage them.

The successful action of a general anaesthetic depends on the predominance if depression over excitation, and the relative invulnerability of the neuronal circuits concerned with the control of respiration and circulation. With any agent that can depress both excitatory and inhibitory synapses indiscriminately, the local balance may be upset in favour of net excitation although, as the anaesthetic level increases, the overall decrease of traffic would be expected to lead to depression.

Anaesthetics affect membranes, not just by dissolving in them, but by producing a change in the physical organization of the membrane. Recent work on the mode of action of general anaesthetics upon cells has revealed a number of correlations between properties of drugs and function of cells but so far no single drug action or group of actions has been shown to be the essential requirement.

THEORIES ON THE ACTION OF GENERAL ANAESTHETICS

Colloid theory

Claude Bernard in the last century considered that narcotics caused a reversible coagulation of cell colloids.

Lipid hypothesis

Meyer (1899) and Overton (1901) independently drew attention to the relationship between anaesthetic potency and the oil-water partition coefficient. Thus it was suggested that the higher the ratio, the more would an anaesthetic dissolve in cell lipids and the more potent would it be. This correlation has been fairly well substantiated.

Protein theories

Binding of anaesthetics to protein is thought to occur to a considerable extent, presumably to non-polar side chains. Altering the protein configuration would affect the membrane activity.

Water hypothesis

Pauling and Miller have suggested that anaesthetic activity follows the interaction between anaesthetic molecules and cell water. Hydrogen bonding could result in the formation of lattices, the anaesthetic molecules being incorporated in the interstices and stabilizing the structure. The existence of these microcrystals could interfere with ionic mobility or enzyme activity and thus interfere with the processes involved in normal function of the cell or its membrane.

Biochemical theories

It is known that under anaesthesia oxygen consumption of the brain is reduced. Narcotics have been shown *in vitro* to depress many enzyme systems. However, cellular narcosis occurs before there is any demonstrable change in oxygen uptake.

KINETICS OF INHALATION ANAESTHESIA

Induction of Anaesthesia

Anaesthesia results from the development of an effective brain anaesthetic partial pressure. To achieve this it is necessary, particularly during induction of anaesthesia, to administer from the anaesthetic apparatus a considerably higher partial pressure than eventually required owing to dilution of anaesthetic gases by air in the tubing of the apparatus and in the patient's respiratory system. The greatest drop in anaesthetic partial pressure from the source of the anaesthetic to the brain occurs between the apparatus and the alveoli.

Concentration in the alveoli is affected by:
· The inspired concentration;
· Alveolar ventilation.

Factors affecting uptake by blood:

Solubility

High blood solubility makes it difficult to achieve a high partial pressure of anaesthetic agent in the plasma on which uptake by the brain cells depends. Less soluble anaesthetics show a relatively fast rise of alveolar and plasma concentration towards inspired concentration, and uptake by the brain is facilitated, resulting in relatively rapid induction of anaesthesia. Nitrous oxide is relatively insoluble, whereas diethyl ether is highly soluble. Halothane occupies a middle position.

Cardiac output

A higher cardiac output increases uptake and lowers alveolar concentration. A low output increases alveolar concentration and speeds induction of anaesthesia.

Venous anaesthetic levels

The greater the difference in partial pressure of the anaesthetic between the alveoli and returning venous blood, the larger is the uptake. Thus uptake is greatest at induction of anaesthesia and complete equilibration takes many hours to achieve. The brain, like the heart and liver, has a high perfusion of blood per unit volume and a relatively short time is therefore required for it to achieve equilibrium with the partial pressure of anaesthetic in arterial blood.

Recovery from anaesthesia

When the administration of an anaesthetic is discontinued, the alveolar partial pressure rapidly falls as a result of respiration. The reversed gradient of partial pressure between the blood and the alveoli now encourages the anaesthetic to pass from the blood to the alveoli whence it is exhaled. The concentration in the blood also falls as redistribution takes place to the body tissues, and this in turn allows the brain to relinquish its relatively generous share of anaesthetic. Its large blood flow, which during induction caused it to receive a high proportion of anaesthetic, now facilitates its clearance. Soluble anaesthetics tend to linger in tissues and blood: the low plasma partial pressure discourages rapid transport of such agents back to the alveoli. Complete elimination from the body tissues may take many hours and accounts for delay in regaining full consciousness. Metabolism plays little part in recovery from inhalation anaesthetics.

KINETICS OF INTRAVENOUS ANAESTHESIA

The intravenous anaesthetics are injected directly into the bloodstream. The concentration of drug reaching the brain depends on dosage, site of injection, speed of injection, concentration of injected solution and rapidity of circulation. Again, those organs with a high blood flow: unit volume ratio (brain, heart, liver) receive a relatively large dose. Similarly, on discontinuing administration the drug is cleared more rapidly from these organs than from body tissues in general. Recovery from anaesthesia is due in the first place to redistribution from the brain, followed by metabolism. Speed of breakdown determines rate of recovery not so much from a minimal sleep dose as from a series of incremental doses, such as are used to maintain anaesthesia with an intravenous agent alone over a prolonged period. In these circumstances an accumulation of drug is gradually built up in the body tissues which may take many hours to be eliminated. A drug which is rapidly metabolized is more suitable for the maintenance of prolonged anaesthesia than one which is relatively slowly broken down if the penalty of a protracted recovery period is to be avoided.

STAGES OF ANAESTHESIA

A brief understanding of the stages of anaesthesia is necessary before con-sideration of individual agents.

Stage 1   Analgesia:
Sensitivity to pain reduced; consciousness and co-operation maintained.

Stage 2   Analgesia:
Patient unconscious, moves spontaneously; reacts physically to stimulus; eyeballs eccentric, moving; pupil often dilated but reacts to light. Most outpatient dental anaesthetics are maintained about lower Stage 2 and upper Stage 3.

Stage 3   Surgical anaesthesia:
Patient immobile — does not move on stimulus; eyeballs centrally fixed; divided into planes marking progressive paralysis of abdominal and thoracic musculature and finally diaphragm. Deep surgical anaesthesia now rarely employed, muscle relaxation where necessary being obtained by neuromuscular blocking agents, e.g. curare-type drugs.

State 4   Respiratory arrest:
Due to central respiratory depression by anaesthetic agent; circulation depressed but still effective; respiration restored by redistribution of agent from brain; life sustained meantime by artificial ventilation of lungs.

These stages were first described with ethyl ether, but despite individual variations they form a useful basis for study of all inhalation anaesthetics. The pattern can also be observed to a certain extent with intravenous anaesthetic agents but there is an important deviation in that severe respiratory depression may be caused before satisfactory surgical anaesthesia (Stage 3) is achieved.

3.2   ADMINISTRATION OF GENERAL ANAESTHETICS

GENERAL CONSIDERATIONS

Even the lightest general anaesthetic may interfere seriously with a patient's airway. During anaesthesia the jaw must be held forward, and the patency of the airway ensured. The airway may be threatened by the presence of secretions and debris in the pharynx; if secretions collect, they must be removed at once with suction by the aid of a laryngoscope.

General anaesthesia in the dental outpatient for the simple extraction of teeth presents particular problems, principally that without the insertion of of an endotracheal tube the operator and the anaesthetist are obliged to share the patient's airway each for a different purpose. They must, therefore, understand one another's difficulties. Furthermore, the absence of an endotracheal tube does not allow efficient protective packing of the pharynx to guard against aspiration of blood or debris into the trachea; reliance must therefore be placed upon the insertion of a McKesson-type gamgee pack placed across the mouth behind the teeth to be extracted in order to curtain off the pharynx. Another difficulty is that control of the depth of anaesthesia may be lost owing to persistent mouth-breathing, especially in purely inhalational techniques. Intravenous anaesthesia is helpful under these circumstances but carries limitations of its own.

To minimize these risks, anaesthesia should be maintained at a plane just deep enough to allow acceptable working conditions, and only simple operations of a duration measured in minutes should be undertaken. If unforeseen difficulties are encountered the operation should be abandoned, to be completed later under local analgesia or endotracheal anaesthesia. Endotracheal anaesthesia may be performed in outpatient dentistry. Usual indications are for the extraction of a number of difficult teeth, or for conservation in a uncooperative child. Intubation of the trachea ensures a patent airway and allows proper pharyngeal packing. The tube may be introduced under inhalation anaesthesia alone or with the help of a neuromuscular blocking agent such as suxamethonium.

PREPARATION OF THE PATIENT

It is of paramount importance that a patient is properly prepared for general anaesthesia or intravenous sedation as follows:

Medical assessment

He must undergo a comprehensive medical assessment with special reference to the cardiovascular and respiratory systems. Careful note is made of any drugs which the patient is taking in case of interaction with the anaesthetic or sedative agent; of particular significance are sedatives and tranquillizers which may increase the depressive effect of an anaesthetic or intravenous sedative. Cardiovascular stability under anaesthesia or sedation may be affected in patients who are on drugs which depress cardiac output or the maintenance of sympathetic tone, e.g. the β-blockers and other antihypertensive agents.

Dental assessment

A full dental examination should be made, if necessary including radiography. This is to determine whether the operation can be performed on an outpatient basis or whether it is advisable to have the patient admitted to hospital. It also allows properly planned treatment to prevent the need for a further general anaesthetic after a short time.

Consent

Informed consent of the patient (or, in the case of those aged under sixteen, the parent or guardian) should be obtained in writing.

Precautions

Every effort is made to ensure an empty stomach. General anaesthesia may induce vomiting and always depresses the protective reflexes of the respiratory tract; inhalation of gastric contents could be fatal. Anaesthetic sessions should be timed for first thing in the morning; otherwise a patient should fast for at least 6hr from the previous meal, which should not be heavy. Bladder and, if possible, bowel, should be empty. Pre-operative sedation prolongs post-anaesthetic recovery and is generally unnecessary. Atropine may be administered intravenously as an anti-sialagogue (adult dose 0.3 mg) but there is little indication for it prior to brief anaesthetics. A responsible adult should accompany the patient and warnings given not to drive or to operate machinery for the rest of the day.

RESUSCITATION

Severe respiratory and cardiovascular depresson are potential hazards of general anaesthesia and sedation. Although they are largely avoidable by careful technique the administrator must possess both the ability and the equipment to deal with these complications. Respiratory depression is managed by maintenance of a clear airway and, if necessary, by positive pressure ventilation of the lungs with oxygen. Cardiovascular collapse is similarly treated, with the patient's head low and legs raised to encourage venous return to the heart and maximum circulation to the brain. Further details on resuscitation techniques are given on pp.195-200.

ANAESTHETIC MACHINES

There are two types of anaesthetic machine in common use for outpatient dental anaesthesia:
    Continuous flow (Boyle, Quantiflex)
    Demand flow (McKesson, Walton, A.E.)

Continuous flow machines

The gases flow continuously, rate of flow being regulated by flowmeters, one for nitrous oxide and the other for oxygen. The combined flow-rate should at least equal the patient's minute volume, i.e. the volume of gas exchanged per minute, calculated by multiplying tidal air (e.g. 500 cc) by respiratory rate (e.g. 18 respirations per minute). This is in order to minimize rebreathing and to avoid excessive retention of CO_2. A satisfactory flow-rate is 9 litres, of which 6 1. is nitrous oxide and 3 1. oxygen, giving a percentage of oxygen of approximately 33 (air is 21% oxygen). The gas mixture passes through a halothane vapouriser. This may be of simple design (e.g. Goldman) but it is of advantage to use a calibrated vapouriser (e.g. the Fluotec) which delivers a constant known percentage of halothane despite variations in gas flow, temperature, etc. It is necessary to incorporate a reservoir bag in the delivery system of a continuous flow apparatus as respiration is an intermittent process rather than a continuous one, and the actual *rate* of flow of gases into the lungs during an inspiration is in excess of 20 litres per minute. Exhalation occurs via a spring-loaded expiratory valve which should be sited as close to the nose as possible in order to reduce dead-space, i.e. the volume of tubing and air passages between the source of fresh gases and the alveoli.

Demand flow machines

Gas flow is triggered by very slight negative pressure produced by the onset of inspiration, provided that the patient is connected in a gas-tight fashion to the delivery system, in this case, the nose-piece. Flow ceases at the end of inspiration, and the expired gases are exhaled through a spring-loaded expiratory valve. As these machines are capable of delivery high rates of gas flow on demand, there is no necessity to have a reservoir bag in the system. The flow-rate of the nitrous oxide and oxygen mixture depends upon the patient's demand; in practice, however, during dental anaesthesia with a nasal mask and open mouth, it is often not possible to ensure a gas-tight connection between patient and machine. The anaesthetist, therefore, sets the machine to deliver gases continuously at a pressure of approximately 5 mm Hg. This may be increased to facilitate nitrous oxide/oxygen induction with the mask held away from the face until consciousness is lost, and also to compensate for air dilution occurring via the open mouth during anaesthesia. Ability to deliver such high rates of flow is the principal advantage of this type of apparatus which has been widely used in dental anaesthesia since the introduction of the McKesson by an American dentist of that name in 1910. Demand-flow machines are generally fitted with the simple Goldman-type halothane vapourizer but calibrated vapourizers are also obtainable. The main disadvantage of the demand flow machine is that it is more complicated and less likely to maintain accuracy than the simpler continuous flow type of apparatus. For this reason, the latter, which is used almost universally in hospital practice, is gaining in popularity also in the dental surgery.

INHALATION ANAESTHESIA

Nitrous Oxide

Drug group: inorganic gas. Formula N_2O.
Physical characteristics: non-irritating; sweet-smelling; non-explosive but supports combustion.

Action

Central nervous system: Nitrous oxide has good analgesic properties in inhaled concentration from 20 to 50 %, but in susceptible patients 50 % may produce unconsciousness. Lack of potency prohibits the establishment of anaesthesia deeper than Stage 2 (Excitement); an increase in concentration above 80 % exposes a patient to hypoxia and is contraindicated.

Respiratory system: Easily inhaled. Little respiratory depression in anaesthetic concentrations.

Cardiovascular system: No direct action on heart. Dilatation of peripheral vessels.

Other systems: No significant effect.

Distribution and excretion
Rapidly absorbed from the alveoli. Does not undergo any chemical reaction in the body and elimination is rapid. There is some deposition in the tissues after prolonged administration but this is not easy to detect clinically.

Toxicity
In absence of hypoxia, essentially nil.

Presentation
Gas cylinder (coloured blue)
Compressed to 750 lb. per square inch.
Stored in liquid state, therefore contents gauge if fitted shows full until cylinder is almost empty.

USE IN OUTPATIENT DENTAL ANAESTHESIA

1   For induction and maintenance of inhalation anaesthesia in association with more potent agents, e.g. halothane.
2   For its analgesic/euphoric properties to facilitate conservation ('Relative Analgesia').

Administration
Light surgical anaesthesia (Stage 3) can usually be satisfactorily maintained by nitrous oxide and oxygen (70 and 30 % approximately) with halothane 1.5 %. The use of 30 % oxygen is a safety factor in the event of any momentary respiratory obstruction which may occur, e.g. during a difficult extraction. Where anaesthesia has been induced by an intravenous agent, nitrous oxide and oxygen alone may be sufficient in short cases to provide

acceptable operating conditions owing to the persisting basal narcotic effects of the intravenous anaesthetic.

Nitrous oxide is used in dentistry also as an analgesic. The patient inhales a mixture of nitrous oxide and oxygen (20 to 50 % nitrous oxide) via a nosepiece. An anaesthetic machine (the Quantiflex) has been designed specifically for the purpose. In practice, the analgesic/euphoric effects of the nitrous oxide should be reinforced by verbal encouragement and local analgesia should also be used in any but the most superficial procedures. The analgesic properties of nitrous oxide are taken advantage of also in the Entonox apparatus which consists of a cylinder containing a 50 % mixture of nitrous oxide and oxygen controlled by a demand valve.

Halothane

Drug group: fluorinated hydrocarbon.
Official preparation: Halothane B.P.
Physical characteristics: colourless liquid; vapour non-irritating on inhalation; sweet-smelling; non-explosive. B.P. = $50.2°C$ at 760 mm Hg.

Action
Central Nervous system: Halothane has relatively poor analgesic properties but surgical anaesthesia (Stage 3) is rapidly established.

Respiratory System: Easily inhaled. Relaxation of muscles of tongue and jaw may cause respiratory obstruction. Bronchodilator. Inhibits secretions. Surgical anaesthesia associated with depression of respiration and raised arterial carbon dioxide tension. Occasional tachypnoea. Overdose causes paralysis of respiratory centre.

Cardiovascular system: Direct myocardial depressant action causes bradycardia, fall in cardiac output and hypotension. Dysrhythmias may occur in presence of raised carbon dioxide tension following depression of sino-auricular node and initiation of ventricular contraction by lower centres in myocardium.

Distribution and Excretion: High tension quickly built up in the brain with rapid induction of anaesthesia. When it is withdrawn reversal of the same process leads to fairly prompt recovery. A small proportion is metabolized in the body and the product excreted in the urine.

Toxicity
Drug interaction: Enhances effects of other respiratory and cardiovascular depressants.

Halothane hepatitis: Suspected but not definitely proven as an entity — possibly a sensitization phenomenon. There should be no objection to the use of halothane for a second or subsequent anaesthetic, within a reasonable number of times, where any other agent which might be substituted has other more important disadvantages.

Presentation
In amber-coloured bottles with thymol 0.01 % added as preservative.

Use in Outpatient Dental Anaesthesia
Anaesthetic of choice in combination with nitrous oxide and oxygen for inhalation anaesthesia in outpatient dentistry because of rapid induction and recovery with minimal after-effects.

Administration
Halothane is the most popular volatile inhalation anaesthetic. It is pleasantly and easily inhaled and its potency facilitates rapid induction of surgical anaesthesia. As an adjuvant to nitrous oxide and oxygen, 1 %-1.5 % maintains light surgical anaesthesia, although up to 4% may be used to establish anaesthesia. Induction with an intravenous agent may have a protective effect against cardiac dysrhythmias.

INTRAVENOUS ANAESTHESIA

Intravenous anaesthetic agents currently used in dental outpatients are:
· the barbiturate, methohexitone sodium (Brietal) — by far the most common
· the eugonol, propanidid (Eponotol), and
· the steroid combination, CT 1341 (Althesin).
   The principal advantage of the intravenous route is the rapid and pleasant induction of anaesthesia. In addition, injection of the anaesthetic directly into the bloodstream, while potentially more dangerous, helps to secure adequate operating conditions speedily in resistant patients.

Methohexitone Sodium

Drug group: barbiturate.
Official preparation: Methohexitone; Methohexital (USA)
Physical characteristics: white crystalline powder, soluble in water to give solutions of pH 10-11.

Action
Central Nervous System: Induces sleep immediately on intravenous injec-

tion. Recovery of consciousness rapid. Minor excitatory phenomena accompany anaesthesia in over 50 % of patients. Restlessness may still persist when anaesthesia is deepened to point of severe respiratory depression. Operating conditions may therefore be poor.

Respiratory System: Relaxation of muscles of tongue and jaw occurs early and may cause upper respiratory obstruction. Increased sensitivity of bronchial and laryngeal musculature. Diminution in rate and depth of respiration. Overdose causes paralysis of respiratory centre.

Cardiovascular System: Depression of vasomoter centre leads to fall in systemic vascular resistance. Normal dosage has little direct effect on the myocardium, and though stroke volume is reduced, blood pressure is well maintained by increase in heart rate and cardiac output. Overdose reduces cardiac output and risks hypotension.

Liver and Kidney: No important effect.

Distribution and Excretion
Level in plasma rises rapidly after injection. Immediately taken up by brain. Readily redistributed to body tissues. Rapid decrease in blood levels is followed by slower fall in keeping with biotransformation. About 15 % metabolized per hour. Recovery of consciousness due to redistribution — less hangover than would be expected from speed of metabolism. Incremental doses have some cumulative effect.

Toxicity
Drug interaction. Enhances effect of other respiratory and cardiovascular depressants. Particular care is indicated in patients with coronary heart disease where even a modest fall in arterial blood pressure may have disproportionate effects on coronary blood flow and cardiac output.

Convulsive movements on induction of anaesthesia.

Histamine release. Severe reactions very rare.

Propanidid

Drug group: eugenol derivative.
Physical characteristics: Yellowish oily solution insoluble in water.
      Dissolved in water-solutble polyoxylated castor oil (Tensid) to make a
      5 % solution (50 mg per ml).

Action
Central Nervous System: Rapid induction of anaesthesia and particularly

speedy recovery. Excitatory phenomena less common than with methohexitone but shortcomings in quality of anaesthesia are similar.

Respiratory System: Jaw relaxation less complete than with methohexitone but respiratory obstruction still possible. Propanidid has a similar effect on respiration except that hyperventilation often occurs on induction.

Cardiovascular System: Similar to methohexitone but there is more evidence of direct cardiac depression in some patients leading to fall in blood pressure.

Liver and Kidney: No important effect.

Distribution and Excretion
Distribution similar to methohexitone. Recovery of consciousness due to redistribution but also rapidly metabolized due to choline-esterase activity. Less cumulative than methohexitone.

Toxicity
Drug interaction. May prolong effect of short-acting depolarising muscle relaxant, suxamethonium. Enhances effects of other respiratory and cardiovascular depressant drugs.
   May cause marked convulsive movements.
   Severe histamine effects reported — skin reactions, bronchospasm, cardiovascular collapse.

CT 1341 (Althesin)

Drug group: steroid
Official preparation: Alphaxalone/alphadolone acetate.
Physical characteristics: severe solubility problems. In recent years Glaxo
   experimented with a pregnane derivative, alphaxolone, which proved to
   be non-irritant at injection site, but practically insoluble in water.
   Solubility improved by using polyoxyethylated castor oil (Cremophore
   E.L.) and further improved by the addition of a derivative of alphaxalone, alphadolone. This mixture of steroids was formulated into the
   injection of 1341 (Althesin)

Action
Central Nervous System: Sleep pleasantly induced within 30 sec. Recovery rapid. After dose of 0.05 mg/Kg full recovery as measured by Rhomberg sign takes 15 min. Restlessness and minor convulsive movements of eyelids and limbs may accompany anaesthesia, but operating conditions probably better than with methohexitone and propanidid.

Respiratory System: Similar to methohexitome but does not cause increased irritability of larynx and bronchi. Apnoea more likely to occur.

Cardiovascular System: Similar to methohexitone. Possible antidysrhythmic — induction with Althesin may be protective against cardiac dysrhythmias during subsequent maintenance of anaesthesia with halothane.

Liver and Kidney: No important effect.

Distribution and Excretion
Following injection highest concentrations found in brain, liver and kidney. Rapidly metabolized by liver and half-life measurable in minutes.

Toxicity
Drug interaction. Enhances effects of other respiratory and cardiovascular depressant drugs.
   Convulsive movements on induction of anaesthesia.
   Mild to severe histamine effects.

CLINICAL APPLICATION

Despite their differing chemical backgrounds methohexitone, propanidid and Althesin have many similarities in their practical use and are best considered together.

Presentation

Methohexitone
Vials containing 100 mg, 500 mg, 2500 mg and 5000 mg of dry powder.

Propanidid
Ampoules containing 500 mg propanidid dissolved in 10 ml polyoxylated castor oil (Tensid).

CT 1341 (Althesin)
Ampules (5 and 10 ml) containing steroids alphaxalone and alphadolone dissolved in an aeqeous vehicle containing 20 % polyoxyethylated castor oil (Cremophore E.L.)

Use in Outpatient Dental Anaesthesia

Methohexitone
For induction, prior to inhalation maintenance for exodontia.

As the sole agent for rapid, simple extractions where the lack of perfect operating conditions is of little consequence.

As the sole agent by an incremental technique maintaining unconsciousness for short conservation procedures. This works well in some patients but neither a perfect airway nor tranquil operating conditions can be guaranteed. Methohexitone has been particularly popular for conservation. Recovery of consciousness is rapid and a patient is soon able to leave the premises. Full recovery may, however, take many hours, and patients must be accompanied home by a responsible adult and advised against driving or operating machinery for the rest of the day.

Propanidid
Best limited to the shortest procedures where rapid recovery is at a premium. Otherwise no advantage over methohexitone and danger of anaphylaxis.

Althesin
Limited but definite usefulness. Induction dose lasts longer than induction dose of methohexitone or propanidid; therefore there is some indication for its use in the longer case, e.g. to cover a procedure lasting several minutes. Also provide smoother transition to inhalation maintenance. Immediate recovery of consciousness perhaps less rapid than with methohexitone but complete recovery no less prompt. Danger of anaphylaxis.

ADMINISTRATION OF INTRAVENOUS ANAESTHETICS

Methohexitone
Powder is made into 1 % (10 mg per ml) or 2 % solution by adding "Water for Injection B.P." (Shelf-life of solution is many weeks but it is not a good habit to store made-up solutions for more than a few days). Induction dose 1.0 mg to 1.75 mg/Kg, e.g. 80-100 mg for a fit adult. A test dose of one-third of expected dose should be given in order to detect unexpected hypersensitivity.

Propanidid
Induction dose 5 mg to 10 mg/Kg. Adult test dose 50 mg. Injected undiluted or with equal volume of normal saline.

Althesin
Induction dose 0.05 ml to 0.07 ml/Kg, e.g. 3-4 ml for fit adult. Inject undiluted. Test dose of 1 ml should be given.

Toxicity

All three drugs induce anaesthesia rapidly and pleasantly, but induction may be accompanied by excitatory phenomena, e.g. mild convulsive movements. Their unaccompanied use should, therefore, be limited to short procedures of comparatively little stimulus and where some movement of the patient does not inconvenience the operator, e.g in simple exodontia.

Despite these shortcomings, some dentists have extended the use of intravenous anaesthesia alone (especially methohexitone) to conservation, using an incremental ultra-light technique, in which an important safety factor is the maintenance of a brisk lash reflex. The method can be successful but it will be understood from the foregoing that there is the constant danger of deepening anaesthesia dangerously in an effort to control restlessness in a difficult patient. The deficiencies of the technique are particularly marked in children who show an even greater reluctance to settle on intravenous agents alone. Respiratory embarrassment during intravenous anaesthesia may be reflected by reduced arterial oxygen tension. It is advisable, therefore, to allow any but the shortest case to breathe oxygen or an oxygen-enriched mixture, e.g. nitrous oxide and oxygen with the latter in a concentration of at least 30%.

Anaphylaxis

Histamine release, with effects varying from skin wheals to bronchospasm and cardiovascular collapse, may follow the injection of propanidid and Althesin. It may occur after the initial injection or the initial dose may sensitize the patient to a subsequent administration. Serious anaphylactic reactions are rare with methohexitone.

Extravenous injection

Extravasation of the solutions is unlikely to cause tissue necrosis. There have been no reports of serious sequelae following inadvertent intra-arterial injection. However, the medial side of the elbow should be avoided as an injection site and methohexitone should not be used in concentrations greater than 2 %.

Venous sequela

Venous thrombosis is unusual and is more likely to occur with propanidid (14 %) and with methohexitone (7 %), particularly if injection is made into a small vein. Methohexitone is occasionally painful when injected into a vein on the back of the hand.

3.5   INTRAVENOUS SEDATION

In contrast to intravenous anaesthesia, sedation aims to maintain consciousness and patient co-operation, with the benefits of greater safety and better operating conditions. There is, however, the risk of unexpected oversedation threatening the airway and producing respiratory depression. It follows that patients attending for sedation should be managed as for general anaesthesia and facilities for resuscitation must be at hand.

Diazepam

Drug group: benzodiazepine (also p.168)
Physical characteristics: dissolved for injection in organic solvents based on propylene glycol.

Action

Central Nervous System: Soporific effect within 1 or 2 min of injection but great individual variation in response to drug. Can produce unconsciousness. Amnesia common. Anti-convulsant (p.189). Reduces skeletal muscle tone by central action.

Respiratory system: Slight depression after moderate dosage.

Cardiovascular System: Some depression of sympathetic tone but little clinical effect if patient is kept in supine position.

Distribution and Excretion

After intravenous injection rapid fall in plasma levels over 20 min. Six to eight hours after injection rise in plasma levels may occur due to enterohepatic recirculation. Concentrations of desmethyldiazepam, a pharmacologically active metabolite rise over the next two days. Cumulative effects of intravenous diazepam probably accounted for also by extensive storage in adipose tissue.

Toxicity

Drug interaction. Depressant effects augmented by other respiratory depressant agents, e.g. intravenous anaesthetics. Restlessness. Prolonged sleepiness and impairment of judgement.

Venous sequelae. The solvent used for diazepam is based on propylene glycol which may give pain on injection into a small vein and can cause thrombosis.

Presentation
Ampoules containing 10 mg diazepam in 2 ml solvent and 20 mg in 4 ml.

Use in Outpatient Dentistry
For sedation by intravenous injection to facilitate conservation and simple surigical procedures under local analgesia. Indicated particularly in excessively nervous patients and for prolonged procedures.

Administration
The patient is prepared as for general anaesthesia. He is placed in the supine position. Atropine sulphate 0.3 mg may be injected intravenously to inhibit salivation. Diazepam is then administered (preferably into a large vein) at a rate of 5 mg per minute until 10 mg has been given, and then at 2.5 mg per minute until the patient becomes sleepy, *but not unconscious.* Local analgesic is now injected and work started. A maximum dose of 20 mg diazepam is not exceeded, even if this fails to produce an obvious effect. Normally, however, 17.5 mg achieves good sedation, accompanied by amnesia. This lasts for about 20 min, after which the patient remains relaxed. He is usually able to leave the premises, accompanied, within 90 min of the initial injection. Success of the method depends on co-operation of the patient and it is not generally suitable for children. Diazepam is unpredictable in its action, probably due to variations in distribution and excretion. A dose of 20 mg may have little apparent immediate action and yet may cause the patient to become very sleepy some hours later. Another effect is that a patient who has apparently made a full recovery may show evidence of irresponsibility for some hours afterwards and it is important to warn both him and the person accompanying him' of the possibility. Diazepam is sometimes used in conjunction with pentazocine (below).

Pentazocine

Drug group: narcotic antagonist (non-D.D.A.) (also p.148)
Physical characteristics: prepared for injection in an isotonic aqueous
  solution.

Action
Central Nervous System: Powerful analgesic with some sedative action causing drowsinesss and dizziness. Addiction reported but very rare (later).

Respiratory System: Depression of respiration, rate more than volume.

Cardiovascular System: Transient fall in cardiac output and in arterial blood pressure, in line with sedative effect. Possibly some direct stimulant action on myocardium.

Distribution and Excretion
After intravenous injection most of the drug rapidly disappears from the bloodstream. About one-fifth of the original dose remains in the tissues 4hr later. Largely metabolized in the body.

Toxicity
Drug interaction. Potentiation of other respiratory depressants, e.g. diazepam. Acute toxicity potentiated by monoamine-oxidase inhibitors. Weakly antagonistic to morphine. Antagonised by naloxone (p.150). May cause vomiting and hallucinations.

Presentation
Ampoules containing 30 and 60 mg pentazocine in 1 and 2 ml respectively.

Use in Outpatient Dentistry
By intravenous injection with diazepam to improve quality of sedation and to give some measure of central analgesia to facilitate conservation and simple surgical procedures under local analgesia. Indicated particularly in excessively nervous patients and for long procedures.

Administration
The technique is a variation of the diazepam sedation. With or without intravenous premedication by atropine 0.3 mg, pentazocine 30 mg is injected undiluted over a period of 2 min. This is followed by incremental diazepam until sedation is produced. Following pentazocine a smaller dose of diazepam will suffice, as both drugs have sedative properties and respiratory depression is more likely. The analgesic effect of pentazocine may permit some simple, less painful procedures to be undertaken without local analgesia. Recovery from an intravenous dose of 30 mg is satisfactory but it should be borne in mind that pentazocine takes some hours to be completely metabolized. Recovery speeded by naloxone 0.2-0.4 mg intravenously.

3.6   LOCAL ANAESTHESIA

Naturally occuring Ester
Cocaine

Esters of benzoic acid
Procaine
Amethocaine

Amides (anilide derivatives)
Lignocaine
Mepivacaine
Prilocaine

A local anaesthetic is a drug which temporarily impedes nerve transmission without depressing consciousness.

It is pedantic to make distinction between analgesia (lack of pain) and anaesthesia (lack of feeling).

Skin and mucous membrane contain numerous nerve endings which perceive touch, temperature and pain. The application of a stimulus, be it mechanical, chemical, thermal or electric, produces an impulse of uniform intensity.

PHYSIOLOGY OF LOCAL ANAESTHETICS

All or None Law

If the stimulus is enough to produce an impulse, that impulse is the same no matter how severe the stimulus. The severity of pain felt is governed by the number of nerve fibres stimulated. The intensity of pain and the patient's response to it vary among individuals and from time to time in the same person.

Pain threshold

The level of stimulation at which pain is felt. This is lowered by fear, apprehension and fatigue. Children have a lower pain threshold than adults and may fail to distinguish between pain and pressure. Conversely, older patients are believed to tolerate pain well.

Latency

Although an isolated nerve fibre can be blocked instantaneously by local anaesthetic, a finite time — usually amounting to minutes — is required for the drug to penetrate and achieve complete block of a mixed nerve bundle. This delay is termed latency and is inversely proportional to anaesthetic concentration.

Recovery time

This exceeds latency by a factor of 2-200 and is directly proportional to concentration so that rapid induction can only be achieved at the expense of slow offset of action.

The response to a local anaesthetic ceases as soon as the drug is removed from its site of action. The most important factor in removal is blood flow which is high in mucous membranes. The action of a local anaesthetic may be prolonged by the addition of a vasoconstrictor such as adrenaline. Thus the more accurately an injection is placed, the shorter the latent period. However, a short delay is advisable after an injection before operative procedures are commenced.

Nerve conduction

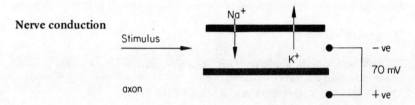

Fig. 3.1 Directions of ionic flux during depolarisation of a stimulated nerve.

Nerve cell cytoplasm contains potassium proteinate: positively charged K^+ and negatively charged Pr^- ions. K^+ can diffuse through the surrounding membrane, Pr^- cannot.

In the extracellular fluid is sodium chloride: positively charged Na^+ and negatively charged Cl^- ions. Cl^- ions are freely diffusible but Na^+ ions are actively extruded from the cell by a mechanism called the sodium pump.

The concentration of K^+ ions inside the cell, 30 times greater than outside, is maintained by an electrical potential keeping the inside of the cell negative to the outside.

The passage of an impulse changes the electrical state of the nerve, the inside becoming +ve in relation to the outside (a potential difference of 70 mV). The membrane becomes permeable to Na^+ ions which move in and K^+ ions flow out (Fig. 3.1). As the impulse passes along the nerve, the cell reverts to its original chemical and electrical state. The change takes only 1.5 miliseconds.

Local anaesthetics act by preventing this migration of ions across the nerve membrane. In low concentration ionic movement is delayed, in greater amounts it is prevented altogether. Nerve fibres of smallest diameter are the most susceptible in the order: sympathetic . . . pain . . . temperature . . . touch . . . motor.

The effectiveness of local anaesthesia depends on:
1   the concentration of local anaesthetic,
2   the solubility of local anaesthetic in water (i.e. extra-cellular fluid) and lipoid (lipoid myelin sheath),
3   and, of course, the accuracy with which the solution is deposited.

USES OF LOCAL ANAESTHESIA

Elimination of pain

For extraction, conservation, minor surgery. Under special circumstances, quite major surgery.

Diagnostic aid

If local anaesthesia abolishes pain, then the cause must be in the area of distribution of the nerve blocked.

Control of haemorrhage

Due to vasoconstrictor content, e.g. prior to surgery, to arrest post-extraction haemorrhage. The local anaesthetic permits suturing while the vasoconstrictor reduces bleeding.

METHODS OF APPLICATION

Topical

Surface anaesthesia by direct application of the drug to skin or mucous membrane.

Infiltration

Deposition of analgesic solution close to the operative site so it can diffuse through soft tissue and alveolar bone.

Regional

Blocking painful impulses by depositing analgesic solution close to a nerve trunk cutting off sensory impulses from the region it supplies.

THE IDEAL LOCAL ANAESTHETIC

Complete local anaesthesia without damage to nerve or tissue
Rapid action
Sufficient duration
Non-toxic
Readily soluble
Stable solution (long shelf-life)
Compatibility with other constituents (e.g. vasoconstrictor)
Easily sterilized
Non-addictive
Isotonic with tissue fluids. Normal pH
Free from undesirable side effect . . . allergy, idiosyncrasy
Inexpensive.

CONSTITUENTS OF LOCAL ANAESTHETICS

Sterile distilled water
Local anaesthetic drug or combination of drugs
Buffers to maintain pH
NaC1 to make solution isotonic
Vasoconstrictor
Preservative to prevent inactivation of vasoconstrictor
Antiseptic

TABLE 3.1 LOCAL ANAESTHETIC DRUGS

Drug	Method	Vasoconstrictor	Contra-indication	Significance
Cocaine	Topical	Powerful vasoconstrictor	Addiction Toxicity Allergy	Historical ENT
Procaine (Novocaine)	2 % injection	Vasodilator Adrenaline 1:80,000	Antagonises sulphonamide. Hypersensitivity	The first widely used synthetic local anaesthetic
Amethocaine	Topical	Vasodilator	Allergy	Prolongs effect of topical anaesthetic containing ligno-caine

Table continued overleaf

Drug	Method	Vasoconstrictor	Contra-indication	Significance
Lignocaine (Xylocaine)	2 % injection and topical	Vasodilator Adrenaline 1:80,000 Felypressin 0.03 iu/ml	Virtually none Toxic reaction to IV injection	The most widely used local anaesthetic today
Mepivacaine (Carbocaine)	2 % injection 3 % injection	Adrenaline 1:80,000 No vasoconstrictor	Similar to Lignocaine	Ultra-short acting For short procedures when adrenaline contraindicated
Prilocaine (Citanest)	3 % injection 4 % injection	Adrenaline 1:300,000 Felypressin 0.03 iu/ml No vasoconstrictor	Patients on high dosage develop methaemoglobin-aemia.	Suitable for longer procedures when adrenaline must be avoided

INDIVIDUAL LOCAL ANAESTHETICS

COCAINE

The numbing effect of the leaves of the coca plant was know to the Incas of Peru, yet the active constituent, cocaine, was not isolated until 1860. The first recorded oral use was by the American surgeon William Stewart Halstead who anaesthetized the inferior dental nerve in 1884. Today it is only used topically, never by injection. Even topically it can cause ischaemic tissue damage, for cocaine is a powerful vasoconstrictor.

Taken orally, the drug stimulates the cerbral cortex, producing a feeling of exhilaration, enabling the user to endure prolonged exhaustion. In excess it may cause hallucination, tremors or convulsions. Finally, it depresses the central nervous system and by depressing the respiratory centre, causes death from respiratory failure. Addiction to this drug results in mental and physical deterioration, the addict becoming a social outcast.

The quest for an improved local anaesthetic resulted in the discovery of the cocaine molecule. Benzoic acid is one of its constituents and many of the esters of benzoic acid were found to have local anaesthetic properties.

Procaine hydrochloride

Procaine hydrochloride is a synthetic ester of benzoic acid. It has no topical value but is used by injection as a 2 % solution. Unlike cocaine, it is a vasodilator and is therefore rapidly dispersed. To prolong its action, a vasoconstrictor is added, e.g. adrenaline. Analgesia lasts 1-2 hr.

All these esters are metabolized by hydrolysis — broken down by esterases in the liver and plasma and excreted in the urine.

Some people develop an allergy to procaine. This applies not only to the patient, but also to the operator. Previous contact with procaine penicillin (depot penicillin) may sensitize a patient to procaine so if there is a history of penicillin allergy, procaine should be avoided.

Procaine inhibits the antibacterial action of sulphonamides. Some oral diabetic preparations are based on the sulphonamide molecule and again procaine can inhibit their action. Hence it must be avoided in these patients.

Amethocaine

Also an ester of benzoic acid, it is ten times more toxic than procaine but finds use in lower concentration as a topical anaesthetic.

Lignocaine

A non-ester, containing an amide linkage. It is unaffected by plasma esterase and is excreted by the kidneys. It is a suitable choice if the patient is allergic to procaine. It may be used topically as a 5 % paste. Otherwise it is used as a 2 % solution and given by injection. Plain lignocaine is available but as it has no vasoconstrictor properties, anaesthesia is transient so adrenaline or felypressin is added. Lignocaine is actually more toxic than procaine but is twice as effective and so can be used in smaller quantities. It lasts longer — 3 hr. Lignocaine is stable with a shelf-life of 2 years. It can be boiled or autoclaved without undergoing change. Hypersensitivity to lignocaine is very rare. It is the most widely used local anaesthetic today.

The maximum safe adult dose is 0.5 mg. For a 2 % solution (with a vasoconstrictor), i.e. 2 mg in 100 ml, the maximum permissible dose would be 25 ml — eleven 2.2 ml cartridges.

Mepivicaine

Also an anilide non-ester. It is not effective topically. It has a weak vasoconstrictor action and may be given as a
3 % solution without adrenaline; or
2 % solution with adrenaline.
It is a short-acting drug (30 min or so) and its main use is for short pro-

cedures when a vasoconstrictor is contra-indicated; it has no other advantage over lignocaine.

Maximum safe adult dose 0.5 mg.

Prilocaine

Another anilide non-ester. It is not a surface anaesthetic. It is less toxic than lignocaine and is rapidly broken down in the liver.

A 3 % solution with adrenaline 1:300,000, or with felypressin 0.03 iu/ml, lasts 1 hr. A 4 % solution without a vasoconstrictor will last ½hr. Patients receiving very high doses of Prilocaine may develop cyanosis due to methaemoglobinaemia. This can be reversed by administering the oxidising agent methylene blue.

Prilocaine with felypressin is a good alternative to lignocaine when the use of adrenaline is contra-indicated.

Maximum safe adult dose 0.6 mg.

USES OF VASOCONSTRICTORS

To reduce blood flow and retard removal of anaesthetic solution, so prolonging its action. Desirable in dentistry but not to be used in end arteries, e.g. finger, where ischaemia may lead to gangrene.

To slow the release of local anaesthetic. Although the drug may be toxic when its concentration exceeds a certain level in the blood, the addition of a vasoconstrictor permits administration of a higher safe total dose. If local anaesthetic is inadvertently injected intravascularly, the vasoconstrictor plays no part in reducing its toxicity.

To allow a smaller volume of local anaesthetic to be used.

To reduce bleeding. If adrenaline or noradrenaline is used for this purpose during a general anaesthetic, ventricular fibrillation may result in a heart sensitized by the general anaesthetic drug. Felypressin may be a suitable alternative, but the anaesthetist must be consulted first.

INDIVIDUAL VASOCONSTRICTORS

Adrenaline

Secreted by the adrenal medulla. Its effect is typified by the 'Flight or Fight' reaction:

· Skin blood vessels constrict, muscle blood vessels (including cardiac muscle) dilate.

· The heart rate increases.

· Blood pressure rises.

These systemic effects do not follow a dental injection unless the solution is injected into a vein. A healthy individual can withstand an intravascular injection, but it is undesirable for a hypertensive patient to have a further elevation of blood pressure. For such cases mepivacaine may be chosen (no vasoconstrictor) or prilocaine with felypressin.

It is important to give an effective local anaesthetic. If the patient feels pain, endogenous adrenaline will be released.

The concentration of adrenaline at 1:80,000 with lignocaine is rather high. Prilocaine with a concentration of adrenaline 1:300,000 is more acceptable.

Noradrenaline

Is released at sympathetic nerve endings. It causes general vasoconstriction but dilatation of the coronary arteries. Its vasoconstrictor effect is half that of adrenaline but patients with hypertension are particulary sensitive to noradrenaline.

There is no justification for using a local anaesthetic containing noradrenaline.

Felypressin

A synthetic preparation related to the posterior pituitary hormone, vasopressin. Vasoconstriction is produced in very low concentrations — 1:2,000,000 (0.03 IU). Felypressin may be used where adrenaline is contra-indicated. It does, however, produce a slight elevation of blood pressure. There is less local ischaemia than with adrenaline and it may be better for anaesthetising teeth with inflamed pulps as there is less likelihood of damaging the pulp's blood supply.

SUMMARY OF COMPLICATIONS

CARDIOVASCULAR

Hypertension
Preferably avoid adrenaline. Use Prilocaine with felypressin or mepivacaine.

Organic heart disease
Minimum local anaesthetic consistent with analgesia. Avoid adrenaline.

Haemorrhagic conditions (e.g. haemophilia)
No injection to avoid risk of haemorrhage.

ENDOCRINE

Thyrotoxicosis
Avoid adrenaline (to which such patients are exceedingly sensitive). Use prilocaine with felypressin or mepivacaine.

Diabetes
Theoretically avoid adrenaline as it is an insulin antagonist. In practice, the patient may be treated as normal.

Steroid therapy
Patients do not tolerate stress. Do not cause pain. Give an adequate local anaesthetic.

CENTRAL NERVOUS SYSTEM DRUGS

Patients taking mono-amine oxidase inhibitors. Noradrenaline released at sympathetic nerve endings is broken down by mono-amine oxidase but the adrenaline used in a local anaesthetic is broken down in the liver. Hence local anaesthetics are not contra-indicated.

Patients taking tricyclic antidepressants. In patients taking these drugs, intravenous injection of adrenaline can cause severe hypertension especially if the patient also has cardiovascular disease. Use prilocaine with felypressin or mepivacaine.

PART 4 · DRUGS IN THE TREATMENT OF COMMON COMPLAINTS

4.1 ANAEMIA

Transfusion
Blood; Plasma expanders

Iron (and desferrioxamine)

Folic acid

Vitamin B$_{12}$
Hydroxycobalamin; Cyanacobalamin

Prednisolone

Anaemia is present when the haemoglobin concentration of whole blood falls below 12 G per 100 ml in males, or 10 G in females. Haemoglobin is confined to red cells and iron is an essential constituent. Anaemia may therefore result from a deficiency of iron or a deficiency of red cells.

Iron and red cells are constantly gained and lost from the body so that the body content of either reflects the dynamic balance between rate of gain and rate of loss. Accordingly, deficiency may result either from diminished gain or accelerated loss. Iron deficiency and red cell deficiency may be the result of the reactions shown below (Fig 4.1)

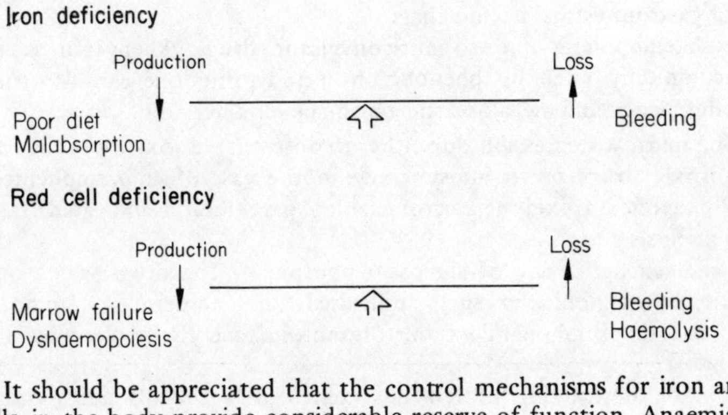

It should be appreciated that the control mechanisms for iron and red cells in the body provide considerable reserve of function. Anaemias will only occur after the reserves (iron stores or marrow capacity) have been exhausted.

Anaemia is a symptom of disease. The manifestations (pallor, breathlessness, tachycardia, fatigue) are fairly constant, but the underlying causes are protean and must be sought. The anaemia may be classified according to aetiology, or morphology of the red cell. For therapeutic purposes, the aetiological classification is of more value:

1   Blood loss. Acute loss simply reduces the number of red cells; chronic loss frequently introduces a factor of iron deficiency.

2   Dyshaemopoiesis (defective red cell maturation) due to defiency of haematinic factors such as iron, vitamin B_{12}, folic acid and vitamin C. Defective cells may either haemoglobinize poorly or haemolyse rapidly. A mixed picture may be present.

3   Marrow (hypoplasia) failure due to infiltrations (e.g. leukaemia), chronic diseases (uraemia, infection, malignant disease), suppression (drugs, chemical poisons, irradiation) diminished stimulus (Addison's disease, myxoedema).

4   Accelerated red cell destruction. (Haemolysis) May occur within the marrow due to failure of cell maturation, in the plasma due to circulating red cell antibodies, or within the reticuloendothelial system due to hypersplenism.

DRUGS AS A CAUSE OF ANAEMIA

Many drugs are the direct cause of anaemia. The common circumstances are:

1   Blood loss due to (a) Gastric erosion due to anti-inflammatory analgesics or corticosteroids, or (b) excessive doses of anticoagulants causing renal or gastrointestinal haemorrhage.

2   Dyshaemopoiesis due to anticonvulsant drugs. Phenytoin is the most commonly cited by phenobarbiton and primidone can also cause folate deficiency and megaloblastic anaemia over a period of years.

3   Bone marrow depression due either to dose-related toxicity in the case of cytotoxic drugs or to idiosyncracy in the case of chloramphenicol, phenylbutazone, troxidone, carbimazole, perchlorate and gold salts.

4   Haemolysis due to:

(a) A red-cell deficiency of glucose-6 phosphate. The drugs which may denature haemoglobin in such individuals are numerous; commonly quoted are the sulphonamides, nitrofurantoin, acetylsalicylic acid, and quinidine.

(b) Immune destruction of red-cells coated with the offending drugs; quinidine and methyldopa are the commonest.

DRUGS USED TO TREAT ANAEMIA

Undoubtedly the drugs most commonly needed to treat anaemias are haematinic factors. However, the administration of iron tablets to every patient presenting with anaemia is quite inappropriate. It cannot be too strongly emphasized that anaemia is merely a symptom of disease; investigation is indicated in every case, both to define the type of anaemia and elucidate its cause.

BLOOD LOSS ANAEMIA

In severe cases of acute loss the immediate danger is of cardiovascular collapse due to loss of circulating volume. Since blood for transfusion must first be cross-matched for compatibility, plasma or plasma substitutes are indicated in the first instance, followed by whole blood when available. The most effective plasma substitutes are the dextrans, high molecular weight polysaccharides which exert a colloid osmotic effect, attracting fluid into the vascular space. Chronic blood loss may be sufficiently mild only to require replacement iron therapy. Higher rates of loss, assuming the cause is untreatable, will necessitate regular transfusion.

DYSHAEMOPOIETIC ANAEMIAS

Defective red cell maturation in this country is most commonly due to deficiency of haematinic factors, caused by dietary lack, pregnancy (increased demand), malabsorption or blood loss. Dietary iron deficiency is not uncommon in the elderly living alone, and menstrual blood loss is the commonest cause of anaemia in women. Pernicious anaemia is due to specific malabsorption of vitamin B_{12}. Malabsorpton syndrome may cause iron and folate deficiencies, and occasionally that of vitamin B_{12}. Vitamin C is necessary for the incorporation of iron into haemoglobin.

Iron

Action
Essential constituent of haemoglobin.

Kinetics
Oral iron is chiefly absorbed in the ferrous state. Pharmaceutical preparations of iron are chiefly the ferrous salts of sulphate, gluconate and fumarate.

The major source of natural iron loss is menstruation which places women of child-bearing age in constant jeopardy of chronic iron deficiency.

Toxicity
1   Gastric upset and nausea are the commonest.
2   Ironificaton of the soft tissues (haemosiderosis) results from chronic parenteral dosage.
3   Acute overdosage is potentially life-threatening, particulary in children.
Oral iron preparations may chelate with tetracyclines, reducing the absorption of both.

Folic Acid

Action
Necessary for metabolism and nucleoprotein synthesis in red cells. Deficiency leads to dysmaturity of the nucleus while cytoplasm continues to accumulate (megaloblastosis). Deficiency may be due to increased demand (pregnancy), malabsorption, and rarely, dietary lack. It may be induced by the excessive demand of marrow malignancies and is sometime seen in patients on long-term anticonvulsant drugs (?due to enzyme induction).

Kinetics
Absorbed from the upper intestine.

Toxicity
None.

Vitamin B_{12} (Cobalamine)

Action
Necessary for the nucleoprotein synthesis in red cells *and* nervous tissue. The deficiency leads to a megaloblastic anaemia, subacute combined degeneration of the spinal cord, peripheral neuropathy, cerebral dysfunction and epithelial changes of mouth and tongue (beef-steak tongue). Folic acid will relieve the anaemia but tends to worsen the nervous manifestations of B_{12} deficiency and for this reason a megaloblastic anaemia must be correctly diagnosed before commencing treatment.

Kinetics
Can only be administered actively by injection. Hydroxycobalamin is strongly plasma-protein bound: cyanacobalamin is less so and therefore

has a significantly shorter half-life. B_{12} must first undergo liver metabolism to become pharmacologically active. It is given every 2-3 months.

Toxicity
B_{12} is non-toxic.

Vitamin C (p.192)
Ascorbic acid deficiency may lead to an iron-resistant anaemia, almost always associated with the signs of scurvy.

HYPOPLASTIC ANAEMIA

Hypoplastic and aplastic anaemia are ideally treated by removal of the cause (e.g. drug). This is ineffective, however, in many cases and regular transfusions of blood are often necessary. Some cases of the idiopathic type of aplastic anaemia (in reality a diagnosis by exclusion and not strictly a type) respond to anabolic steroids.

HAEMOLYTIC ANAEMIAS

Where haemolytic anaemia is symptomatic of another treatable disease the prognosis is good. Corticosteroid drugs (prednisolone chiefly, (p.156) may offer symptomatic benefit in the following situations:
1 Auto-immune haemolytic disease.
2 Immune haemolysis during relapses of myelomatosis and lymphatic leukaemia.
3 Hereditary non-spherocytic anaemias.
  Where a drug is the suspected cause of haemolysis, it should of course be withdrawn.

4.2 ANGINA

Glyceryl trinitrate (and long-acting analogues)

β-adrenoceptor blockers
Propranolol; Oxprenolol

Anxiolytic agents

Oxygen

Angina pectoris (literally strangling of the chest) is the symptom experienced when the heart muscle becomes critically short of oxygen. The capacity of the myocardium for anaerobic metabolism is slight; if the oxygen supply is critically reduced, or the demand increased, ischaemic heart pain may result. Although angina most commonly results from decreased perfusion of blood (through narrowing of coronary vessels) factors which reduce blood oxygen tension such as lung disease may be contributory.

Coronary atheroma is essentially irreversible so that most drug therapy is aimed at reducing myocardial oxygen consumption.

The most important determinants of myocardial oxygen consumption are:

1   Tension (muscle fibre tension).
2   Contractility (strength of contraction).

Tension increases if the ventricle dilates (the fibres are stretched) and this is usually due to heart failure. Contractility rises:

1   As a natural response to increasing tension (Starling's law of the heart), or
2   As a direct effect of adrenergic stimulation (i.e. emotion, exercise).

Drugs effective in angina either reduce tension or reduce contractitility. (They do not, as was once thought, dilate coronary vessels; anoxia itself causes maximum dilatation.) Anti-anginal drugs are discussed with these considerations in mind.

NITRITES AND NITRATES

Inorganic nitrites and nitrates and organic nitrates dilate smooth muscle by a direct effect which is incompletely understood. The effect of sublingually administered glyceryl trinitrate (GTN, the most commonly used of the group) is dominated by dilatation of the systemic veins. These veins can contain up to 80 % of the circulating blood volume and their dilatation results in a rapid fall in venous return to the heart. The filling volume of the ventricles fall as a result of which there is a primary fall in tension (and blood pressure.) A reflex increase in sympathetic activity tends to increase contractility, an unwanted and counteractive effect.

OTHER NITRITES AND NITRATES

1   Amylnitrite is inconvenient (it has to be inhaled), expensive and unpleasant (can cause severe headache).
2   Long-acting nitrates

(a) Pentaerythritol tetranitrate is one of a group of similar drugs marketed for the prevention of anginal attacks. None has proved effective. All are swallowed and thus absorbed into the portal circulation; much of their activity is lost through liver metabolism.

(b) Sustained action glyceryl trinitrate. Pharmacologically active but only used in the most refractory cases owing to common side effects.

KINETICS

The onset of action of GTN is more rapid, and effect much greater if absorbed from the oral rather than gastric mucosa. It's often more useful therapeutically if taken in anticipation of events known to provoke angina.

TOXICITY

1   Blood vessel dilatation: throbbing headache and postural fall in B.P. (dizziness, weakness, syncope).

2   Drug rash.

3   Methaemoglobinaemia: the nitrite ion readily oxidises haemoglobin to methaemoglobin which impairs the oxygen carrying capacity of the blood. Organic nitrates do not oxidise haemoglobin.

TOLERANCE

Tolerance and cross-tolerance are common; thus the continued use of pentaerythritol tetranitrate to prevent angina may reduce sensitivity to glyceryl trinitrate when needed in the acute attack.

β-ADRENOCEPTOR BLOCKING DRUGS (p.93)

The effect of propranolol in reducing myocardial oxygen consumption derives from its β-blocking properties and not from its local anaesthetic action. The response is proportional to the reduction in contractility which follows its administration. It is essential to conserve contractility in heart failure so that β-blocking drugs are contra-indicated in this condition.

In cases of coronary narrowing without heart failure, angina attacks are commonly precipitated by exercise or emotion. Both are associated with rising adrenergic activity which increases myocardial contractility. β-blockade is often very successful in the prophylaxis of angina. Propranolol

is also effective in blocking the reflex increase in contractility which
follows the use of glyceryl trinitrate. (see above) In this respect, the two
are synergistic; in practice GTN tablets are less frequently required by
those patients also taking β-adrenoceptor blockers, and when used tend to
be more effective.
Oxprenolol is less potent than propranolol (potency is important where
action depends on competitive antagonism) but lacks significant local
anaesthetic (depressant) effect.

KINETICS

All oral preparations are rapidly absorbed. Metabolism of β-adrenoceptor
blockers is discussed on page 94.

ANXIOLYTIC DRUGS (p.166)

The rise in adrenergic activity which accompanies exercise is physiological.
However, autonomic activity which accompanies chronic anxiety is the
source of many distressing symptoms — tremor, bowel disturbance,
sweating, increased muscle tone, palpitation, and in those predisposed by
coronary narrowing, angina. Most of these symptoms will respond to
β-blockade by propranolol but there is often a place for the trial of a mild
anxiolytic drug such as diazepam; if successful in treating the anxiety,
diazepam will accordingly reduce the associated autonomic hyperactivity.

OXYGEN

In a state of protracted angina, particularly if associated with respiratory
disease or anaemia, oxygen therapy is a rational adjunct to drug therapy.
Precautions to be observed in applying oxygen to patients with chronic
obstructive airways disease are discussed on page 87.

4.3   HYPERTENSION

Chronic hypertension
Thiazide diuretics
    Chlorthalidone
β-adrenoceptor blockers
    Propranolol
    Oxprenolol

α-Methyldopa
Clonidine
Reserpine
Post-ganglionic adrenergic neurone blockers
    Guanethidine
    Bethanidine
    Debrisoquine
    The above list ranks anti-hypertensive drugs in the order in which they
are often exhibited in the treatment of increasingly severe hypertension.
Individual preferences commonly prevail among physicians. Reserpine is
less frequently used today.

Hypertensive emergency
Diazoxide
Pentolinium tartrate

In broad terms the BP is dependent upon cardiac output and peripheral
resistance:

$$BP \times C.O. \times P.R.$$

These in turn are dependent on other factors. Cardiac output has two components — stroke volume and heart rate. Stroke volume matches venous
return to the heart so that a rise in BP can be expected to result from
excessive blood volume which is usually caused by salt-retention. Heart
rate is under autonomic control, both nervous (predominantly β adrenergic
receptors) and hormonal (circulating adrenaline). Peripheral resistance is
also modulated by autonomic influences and tends to rise with age and
atherosclerosis. Finally nervous reflexes are present throughout the body
to counteract sudden changes in pressure such as may otherwise occur in
rising from a chair (tachycardia and vasoconstriction) or from an accidental
intravenous injection of a pure vasoconstrictor (venous dilatation and
cardiac slowing).
    Blood pressure is intimately related to kidney function; specialized
kidney cells sense blood volume and secrete renin which indirectly
stimulates the adreno-cortical production of aldosterone, a powerful
salt-retaining hormone. Renin may also cause profound peripheral vasoconstriction. Inappropriately high plasma renin values are found in cases of
accelerated (malignant) hypertension associated with vascular necrosis of
the kidneys.
    It is now accepted that the initial abnormality in hypertension is an
elevated cardiac output; over a period of time the output falls towards

normal at the expense of a rising peripheral resistance. Causes of the initial rise in output could be an increase in adrenergic drive to the heart, or rise in blood volume (secondary to changes in sodium balance.) Hypertension is frequently defined as a BP exceeding 120/90. However, a progressive rise in blood pressure is a physiological response to ageing so that 160/120 may be quite acceptable in old age. In a minority of hypertensives, a single specific and reversible cause may be found such as unilateral renal disease or endocrine tumour. The vast majority of cases, however, are idiopathic and treatment is symptomatic, aimed at reducing either cardiac output or peripheral resistance. Finally, environmental factors such as sodium intake, weight, stress and life style should not be omitted when considering the management of hypertension.

DRUG-INDUCED HYPERTENSION

Many drugs are capable of causing hypertension either by raising blood volume (oestrogens, carbenoxolone) by increasing peripheral resistance (catecholamines such as noradrenaline, amphetamines) or by interaction (discussed more fully on p.74).

TREATMENT OF HYPERTENSION

Drugs are aimed at reducing either cardiac output or peripheral resistance. Sympathetic pathways influence both components of blood pressure so that antihypertensive drugs frequently exert a dual action.

DRUGS ACTING PRINCIPALLY TO REDUCE CARDIAC OUTPUT

Stroke volume

Thiazide diuretics. Although their action is primarily to reduce blood volume, thiazides continue to exert a hypotensive effect by direct reduction of peripheral resistance. Alone, their action is weak; however the synergism obtained from combination with other anti-hypertensive agents is often very valuable therapeutically. Thiazides are less likely to cause hypokalaemia in this setting than in the treatment of oedema (p.80).

Heart rate

β-adrenergic blockers. All β-blockers reduce heart rate. Some, such as propranolol also depress contractility and reduce stroke volume. Vascular reflexes are maintained so that postural drops in blood pressure are not usually experienced. β-blockers are particularly useful when angina complicates hypertension. They are discussed more fully on p.93.

Note

Drugs which reduce cardiac output are liable to cause a rise in plasma renin so that increased peripheral resistance may be the price paid for a drop in cardiac output. This response probably accounts for the considerable synergism frequently obtained by combining two drugs with different actions.

DRUGS ACTING PRINCIPALLY TO REDUCE PERIPHERAL RESISTANCE

Peripheral resistance is under sympathetic nervous control, both reflex and central. Drugs which act on peripheral nerves frequently block vascular reflexes and cause postural fainting. Those which act centrally (on the hypothalamic sympathetic outflow) are usually free of postural hypotension.

Predominantly central action

Tranquillizers
Stress is a cause of chronic as well as acute elevations in blood pressure. Where appropriate, mild tranquillizers such as diazepam may reduce the pressure.

Clonidine
Has a predominantly central effect upon sympathetic outflow and preserved postural reflexes.
    Toxicity: dry mouth, sedation and depression.

Reserpine
Derived from the alkaloids of Benth (Rauwolfia Serpentina) and little used to-day on account of side-effects. It depletes stores of sympathetic amines in brain, blood vessels and adrenal medulla by deamination.
    Toxicity: Severe, sometimes suicidal depression. Diarrhoea, weight gain and fluid retention may occur.

Predominantly Peripheral action

a—Methyldopa

Blocks the synthesis of noradrenaline by peripheral sympathetic nerve endings. Vascular reflexes are generally well-preserved although tone is reduced.

Toxicity:
1 Sedation and mild depression (a central action is invoked).
2 Immune haemolytic anaemia. 20 % of patients develop red-cell antibodies but only a small number become clinically anaemic. More important the antibodies interfere with cross-matching of blood.
3 Weight gain and sodium retention; nasal stuffiness.

Post-ganglionic adrenergic neurone-blockers

The 'parent' drug is guanethidine, which has a slow onset of action and long t½. More recent additions to the group are more rapid in action. All of them block the nerves subserving vascular reflexes but because their action is post-ganglionic, they do not affect the adrenal gland output of adrenaline and noradrenaline. Lack of sympathetic stimulation leaves the blood vessel adrenoceptors highly sensitive to circulating pressor substances.

Toxicity:
1 Hypotension on change of posture or following exercise is frequently very troublesome.
2 Weakness, sedation and depression.
3 Diarrhoea and failure of ejaculation.

Bethanidine and debrisoquine are alternative drugs offering greater flexibility.

Diazoxide

A thiazide-related drug without diuretic properties which retains the property of relaxing vascular muscle, and given intravenously during hypertensive crises usually produces a smooth and rapid fall in BP.

DRUG INTERACTIONS WITH ANTIHYPERTENSIVE AGENTS

Sympathomimetic amines

Drugs such as amphetamine, isoprenaline, metaraminol and adrenaline can displace post-ganglionic adrenergic neurone blockers from their site of action and reverse their antihypertensive effect. In addition, the blocking drugs may sensitize adrenoceptors to the action of circulating pressor amines. Many cold-cures and cough mixtures contain significant quantities of such pressor amines. It is unlikely that adrenaline in the concentrations used in dentistry, will produce such effects.

Tricyclic antidepressant

Tricyclic drugs block the amine pump normally responsible for the uptake by nerve endings of adrenergic neurone blocking drugs. The result is either negation or reversal of the antihypertensive's action; serious *rises* in blood pressure can result.

Many antihypertensive drugs cause depression so that as a group, hypertensive patients are more than randomly exposed to the use of antidepressant drugs.

The interaction of tricyclic antidepressants with methyldopa is contentious; antagonism of clonidine has been reported.

Phenothiazines

Chlorpromazine has intrinsic a-blocking (hypotensive) activity but in combination with adrenergic neurone blockers may antagonize their action.

Fluid retaining drugs

Carbenoxolone, Indomethacin, Phenylbutazone and Corticosteroids all have sodium and fluid retaining properties which by raising the blood volume can antagonize the action of antihypertensive agents.

Drugs potentiating antihypertensive agents

1 Diuretics may cause significant falls in blood volume, particularly when first introduced.
2 Phenothiazines, MAO inhibitors and tricyclic antidepressants can all cause major falls in BP (in the absence of adrenergic neurone blockers).

GENERAL ANAESTHESIA AND ANTIHYPERTENSIVE DRUGS

The major fear is the induction of irreversible hypotension under anaesthesia. The hypotensive action of diuretics, reserpine, methyldopa and adrenergic neurone blockers can be reversed by direct acting sympathomimetic drugs such as isoprenaline (β-stimulant) or metaraminol (α-stimulant).

4.4   HEART FAILURE

Digoxin

Aminophylline

Diuretics (Saluretics)

Oxygen (see Respiratory disorders)

Morphine (see Pain)

PHYSIOLOGY OF THE CIRCULATION

The heart works as two separate pumps: the stronger of the the the two, the left ventricle, pumps blood at high pressure through the organs of the body. The capillaries in these organs offer a high resistance so that a substantial pressure drop occurs as blood passes through them to the venous side of the circulation. Before returning to the left ventricle, blood has to traverse the lung capillaries which offer further resistance to its flow. An auxiliary pump, the right ventricle, is situated just before the lungs and steps up the blood pressure enough to overcome pulmonary resistance. The circulation is therefore a single closed circuit containing two functionally separate pumps (Fig. 4.2).

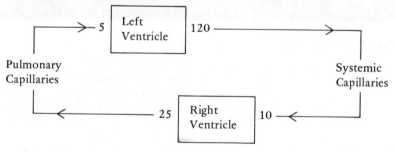

PUMP FAILURE AND SALT RETENTION

If the major pump (left ventricle) fails while the minor continues to pump normally, the disparity in output will lead to a build-up of pressure in the pulmonary capillaries and a leakage of plasma into the alveoli; the result is pulmonary oedema and narrowing of the airways. This situation is common following an acute infarction of the left ventricle (heart attack). With a damaged pump whose output is falling, the entire circulation naturally slows and the blood pressure within the *systemic* capillaries falls. Systemic oedema is characteristic of chronic heart failure. Yet oedema only occurs where capillary pressure is abnormally high. The explanation lies in the kidney's reflex response to a falling perfusion pressure. Apart from a general tendency of the kidney to reabsorb sodium when BP falls, specialized cells indirectly stimulate the adrenal glands to secrete a powerful salt-retaining hormone called aldosterone. This hormone causes reabsorption into the circulation of salt (and an equivalent amount of water) which might normally be lost in the urine. The overall result is an expansion of blood volume, rise in capillary pressure and oedema of the surrounding tissues (Fig. 4.3).

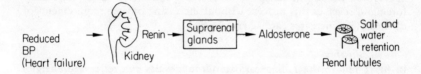

There are three major sites in this process at which therapeutic agents can be aimed:
1   Pump failure — digoxin, aminophylline
2   The body excess of salt and water — diuretic agents
3   The specific renal mechanism for salt retention — aldosterone antagonists.

PUMP FAILURE

DIGOXIN

Derivation. Digoxin has been known to medicine for centuries and is one of a group of drugs of mainly plant origin which have a specific and powerful effect on cardiac muscle. The active constituents of these drugs are known as cardiac glycosides because each has a structure containing molecules of sugar. Digoxin, the mostly widely used today, is one of three such glycosides obtained from the fox-glove (*Digitalis lanata*). Nowadays digoxin is prepared semisynthetically and is more predictable in its effects than the crude plant extract.

Cardiac effects of digoxin

1   Increase in force of contraction.
2   Depression of conducting tissue — principally an increase in refractory period of the a-v node.
3   Vagal effect: (a) Decrease in atrial refractory period; (b) Delay in a-v conduction (as above).
4   Increased myocardial excitability.

Increased contraction
This is the primary effect of digoxin on the heart and occurs independently of physiological control. Contractility is normally controlled through adrenergic influence (sympathetic nervous system and circulating adrenaline) and through an intrinsic mechanism whereby the force of the contraction automatically increases as the load imposed on the ventricle (tension) rises. Both mechanisms have limits beyond which the ventricle dilates and its output falls, i.e. it fails. Digoxin increases the contractile force and reverses this process without increasing oxygen requirements of the heart; i.e. increases cardiac efficiency.

Cardiac Slowing
In heart failure the falling cardiac output results in a reflex (adrenergic) speeding up of the heart. By improving cardiac output digoxin will therefore reduce heart rate.

Kinetics

Digoxin is well-absorbed orally. It is partly bound to plasma proteins and has a normal half-life of about 48hr, accounting for its tendency to be cumulative. It is not significantly metabolized, but is excreted largely unchanged by simple filtration through the renal glomeruli. Glomerular filtration rate (reflected in serum urea and creatinine levels) has therefore a very important influence on the plasma level of digoxin.

Toxicity

1   Systemic effects. Most common are the gastro-intestinal symptoms of anorexia, nausea, vomiting and bowel disturbance.
2   Cardiac effects. Generally speaking, healthy hearts respond to toxicity with heart block and damaged hearts with changes in rhythm.
3   Potentiation by low serum potassium level. In practice, one of the common causes of digoxin toxicity is hypokalaemia, commonly resulting

from the concurrent use of a potassium-losing diuretic with inadequate potassium supplementation.

The dose of digoxin must be reduced in the presence of renal failure. The elderly are relatively intolerant to the drug.

AMINOPHYLLINE (THEOPHYLLINE + ETHYLENE DIAMINE)

The specific actions of aminophylline useful in cardiac failure are:
1 Cardiac stimulant action
2 Bronchodilator effect
3 Diuretic effect

The cardiac stimulant effect is direct and immediate after i.v. administration and is synergistic with that of digoxin. Cardiac output is increased.

Kinetics

Aminophylline is well absorbed orally but its use via this route is limited by gastric irritation. It is absorbed slowly when given rectally, the usual route, and may be given i.v.

Toxicity

1 Rapid i.v. injection may cause an acute fall in blood pressure. Tachycarida and ectopic rhythms may accompany even slow injection.
2 Overdosage may lead (in addition to the above) to excitement, delirium and even convulsions.

SALT RETENTION

From its Greek derivation, the word diuretic means urine promoting agent. However, these drugs primarily cause a salt diuresis and are more accurately termed saluretics.

PHYSIOLOGY OF SODIUM EXCRETION

Sodium and water filtered freely by the kidney glomeruli and about

99.5 % is reabsorbed by the tubules at three principal sites:
1   Proximal tubule — about 60 % of filtered sodium is reabsorbed with an
equivalent amount of water.
2   Loop of Henle — Sodium *alone* is avidly reabsorbed from the
ascending limb and passes into the descending (proximal) limb producing
highly-concentrated fluid in and around the tip-of the loop (counter-
current multiplier, Khun 1942).
3   Distal tubules — Sodium is reabsorbed, again without water, further
diluting the urine. At the near end of the distal tubule, sodium is reabsorbed
independently; at the far end, reabsorption involves exchange for H^+ and
K^+ ions from the tissue fluid and plasma.

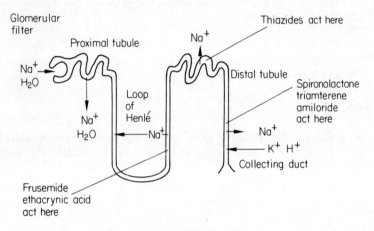

Sites of action of diuretics

(saluretics)

Diuretics act in one of two ways:

*(a) By presenting the far end of the distal tubules with large amounts of
sodium so that their capacity to reabsorb it is exceeded.*
Such diuretics are potassium-losing:
1   Frusemide and ethacrynic acid prevent sodium reabsorption from the
ascending loop of Henle and destroy the counter-current mechanism. By
this means large amounts of sodium are retained in the urine, accounting
for the high potency of these saluretics.
2   Thiazide diuretics act principally on the distal convoluted tubule, at its
near end, preventing reabsorption of sodium alone.
       Presented with an increased sodium load, the sodium reabsorbing
mechanism at the far end of the distal tubule is stressed beyond its limits
and there will be a considerable loss of potassium and hydrogen ions.

Overall result: Salt diuresis with hypokalaemic, hypochloraemic, alkalosis.
Note: Therè are a number of commercially-produced combined preparations which contain a thiazide and potassium supplement in fixed dosage. They have two major disadvantages:
1 The potassium content may be insufficient.
2 Simultaneous administration of the two drugs is inefficient.

(b) By preventing sodium/potassium-hydrogen exchange at the far end of the distal tubules
Such diuretics are potassium-conserving.
Spironolactone. It will be remembered that the salt-retaining mechanism operating in congestive heart failure involves production of excess aldosterone which facilitates sodium/potassium-hydrogen exchange. This action is directly antagonized by Spironolactone. The important practical points to grasp are:
1 That Spironolactone in itself is a weak diuretic (influencing a mechanism which accounts for a relatively small percentage of total sodium normally reabsorbed).
2 That in combination with a thiazide or frusemide it is highly synergistic, facilitating their maximum effect.
3 That alone it leads to net *retention* of potassium. Triamterene and Amiloride are similar to spironolactone.

COMPARATIVE PHARMACOKINETICS

All the above mentioned preparations are readily absorbed after oral administration. Frusemide is the most rapidly acting (an effect can be observed within 30 minutes) and spironolactone is the slowest, taking some days to achieve maximum effect. Frusemide has a very brief duration of action; the majority of thiazides are excreted within 3-6 hours but some (e.g. chlorthalidone) have a longer duration of action (18-24 hours) related to their slower rate of excretion. The majority of diuretics are excreted by the kidney.

Toxicity

Hypokalaemia
Frusemide, ethacrynic acid and the thiazides may lead to severe hypokalaemia if used without adequate potassium supplements. The attendant dangers are muscular weakness, digitalis sensitivity and cardiac dysrhythmias; characteristic ECG changes occur. Despite such chemical changes,

these diuretics will continue to act so that, if carelessly used, severe electrolyte disturbances can result.

Hyperkalaemia
The use of potassium conserving diuretics may result in hyperkalaemia, particularly in renal failure, where potassium excretion is already reduced. Cardiac standstill may result.

Hyperuricaemia and hyperglycaemia
Frusemide, ethacrynic acid and the thiazides interfere with uric acid excretion. Clinical gout sometimes results. The same diuretics reduce insulin secretion and, in those predisposed, clinical diabetes mellitus may ensue.

Acute saline depletion
Excessive dosage of the more potent diuretics may lead to an acute loss of circulating volume resulting in lethargy and a fall in blood pressure, usually most noticeable when the patient stands up — postural hypotension.

4.5 RESPIRATORY DISEASE

1 Obstructive airways disease — acute and chronic
Sodium cromoglycate
β-adrenoceptor-stimulants

Salbutamol
Terbutaline Sulphate
Isoprenaline
Orciprenaline
Adrenaline

Theophyllines

Aminophylline
Choline theophyllinate

Corticosteroids

Hydrocortisone
Beclomethasone
Prednisolone

Antibiotics

Oxygen

2 Cough
Expectorants

Proprietory and BPC mixtures

Mucolytics   Bromhexine
                                    Acetylcysteine

Suppressants   Demulcents
                                    Antihistamines
                                    Codeine phosphate
                                    Pholcodeine
                                    Methadone

3 Upper respiratory (nasal) congestion
Ephedrine

4 Respiratory depression
Nikethamide

COMMON PATHOLOGIES

Obstructive airways disease
Cough
Upper respiratory congestion
Respiratory depression

PHYSIOLOGY OF LUNG FUNCTION

The lungs perform the function of gas exchange. Without oxygen the patient becomes cyanosed and tissue function (particularly cerebral function) deteriorates rapidly. Unable to excrete carbon dioxide the patient becomes drowsy and tremulous; fatal coma may ensue.

Essential to lung function are (a) ventilation, and (b) alveolar respiration (gas exchange). Ventilation is a mechanical process requiring the integrity of brain stem (respiratory centre), nervous connections, muscles (diaphragm, intercostal muscles), lung parenchyma (elastic tissue) and the patency of airways. Respiration on the other hand is a passive phenomenon of gas diffusion dependent upon the integrity of the alveolar membranes and blood supply to them.

Lung disease may affect either ventilation or respiration (or both). However, the exchange of gases is affected differently in either case. Failure of ventilation affects the passage of CO_2 out of the lungs as much as it does oxygen into them, and a combined hypercapnia/anoxemia results. On the other hand, CO_2 diffuses 40 times more rapidly than oxygen and before alveolar disease can be serious enough to produce signs of hypercapnia, the patient will be dead through anoxia. Pure alveolar disease (e.g. fibrosing alveolitis) therefore results in anoxia without hypercapnia. In fact the reflex tachypnoea which usually accompanies alveolar disease causes hyperventilation and the Co_2 tension in the blood commonly *falls*. Blood gas analysis can therefore help to define the type of lung disease.

The commonest cause of ventilatory failure is obstructive airways disease. This may be reversible (e.g acute allergic asthma) or essentially irreversible (e.g. chronic bronchitis). The distinction is clinically and therapeutically important. Acute asthma is the result of sudden constriction of bronchial smooth muscle and usually responds rapidly to appropriate therapy. Chronic bronchitis leaves the airways scarred and permanently narrowed through repeated or chronic infection. In exacerbations, which are usually due to infection by low-grade respiratory pathogens, large volumes of purulent sputum are produced which further occlude the airways and since this situation is generally treatable, a reversable element can be said to be present. In contrast to acute asthma, however, full patency of the airways can never be restoed in chronic bronchitis and the essential factor in therapy is to prevent infection getting a hold.

THE USE OF DRUGS IN ACUTE OBSTRUCTIVE AIRWAYS DISEASE

Asthma, in those predisposed, is commonly due to allergy, infection or to no apparent cause (idiopathic). Sometimes emotional status is important. It seems probable that infection can trigger an allergic response in susceptible patients.

The allergic response in asthma is due to the break-up of mast cells in the bronchial submucosa with the release of smooth-muscle stimulants such as histamine, bradykinins and S-R-S (slow reacting substances). Susceptible individuals possess reagin, an antibody which is fixed to the lining of the bronchi; it is the interaction of allergen and antibody which initiates disintegration of the mast cells.

Where an allergen can be identified, avoidance is important and a desensitization course may be valuable.

Prophylaxis

Antihistamines
Generally ineffective.

Sodium cromoglycate
This revolutionary new drug, which is taken by inhalation, has been shown to prevent the break up of mast cells consequent upon allergen-reagin com-

bination. It is effective in both "allergic" and "infective" asthmatics. It is not absorbed and is non-toxic.

Corticosteroids (see p.156)

The glucocorticoids such as prednisolone have powerful anti-inflammatory properties and tend to synergise the effects of β-adrenergic stimulants. However their severe side-effects preclude their long-term use in all but the most severe relapsing asthmatics. The kinetics and toxicity of corticosteroids are discussed elsewhere (p.159). The dentist should take care to increase the dose of steroids prior to a surgical procedure, and ensure that hydrocortisone injections are to hand.

Beclomethasone

A more recent development has been the introduction of a steroid inhalant, beclomethasone. It has been claimed (and justifiably it seems) that the drug has a mainly local action and is effective in the prophylaxis of severe asthma without systemic toxicity.

The acute attack

Sodium cromoglycate is a prophylactic only and is *ineffective* in the acute attack.

β-adrenoceptor stimulants

β-stimulation of bronchial smooth muscle causes dilatation. A number of β-stimulants are in use but only Salbutamol and Terbutaline offer any degree of broncho-selectivity (β_2-receptors). Such drugs are most effective if delivered as a fine mist (aerosol); the efficiency of such administration is naturally reduced during acute bronchospasm. Adrenaline (1 ml of 1:1000) is given by subcutaneous injection and its rapidity of action may be life-saving.

Isoprenaline A pure β-stimulant and readily absorbed from an aerosol. It is not bronchoselective and the cardiovascular response to even small quantities is tachycardia, palpitation, headache and skin flushing (peripheral vasodilatation).

Toxicity. Exaggerated CVS responses. In those predisposed (e.g. ischaemic heart disease) isoprenaline may cause anginal pain, weakness, acute dysrhythmia or occasionally cardiac arrest if the myocardium is subjected to a sudden load.

Orciprenaline

Like isoprenaline, is a non-selective β-stimulant. It is longer acting than isoprenaline. Usually given by aerosol.

Salbutamol and Terbutaline sulphate
Both are selective β_2 stimulants with only slight cardiovascular effects. Tremor of skeletal muscle, common to all β-stimulant drugs can occur in therapeutic dosage. May be given by aerosol, tablet or injection.

Note on the use of sympathomimetic aerosols

'While a casual relationship between increased use of pressurized aerosol preparations and the epidemic of asthma deaths has not been conclusively established, the evidence is so strong that every care should be taken to avoid *excessive* (our emphasis) use of aerosols for the treatment of asthma in the future. . . nevertheless aerosols properly used are of considerable value in the treatment of asthma.'

This extract of a letter from the Scottish Home and Health Department dated August 1973 followed a tragic rise in asthma deaths which accompanied the widespread introduction of isoprenaline and related drugs in pressurised aerosols between 1961 and 66. The rise in death rates occurred chiefly in young asthmatics and the mortality curves follow very closely the sales of pressurized aerosols. Since 1967, when warnings were intimated to practitioners directly and through the medical journals, the mortality rates fell rapidly as did the sales of aerosols. The relationship cannot be ignored and reflects the ease with which, even in modern times, apparently simple drugs can kill.

Adrenaline
The powerful β-stimulant effect of subcutaneous adrenaline is useful in the acute asthmatic attack. It is non-selective and also has a-adrenergic (vasoconstrictive) effects.

Toxicity: Following s.c. administration, palpitation, extrasystoles and hypertension are common; prolonged cardiac dysrhythmias sometimes occur. It should never be given i.v. except in extreme situation (e.g. anaphylaxis).

Theophyllines

Aminophylline
A potent bronchodilator following intravenous injection.
Kinetics: (p.79). It is given by slow (15 min) i.v. injection of a dilute solution (250 mg in 10 ml).
Toxicity: Mainly cardiovascular. Palpitation is common.

Choline theophyllinate
An orally effective theophyllinate which lacks the gastric irritation associated with aminophylline.

THE USE OF DRUGS IN CHRONIC OBSTRUCTIVE AIRWAYS DISEASE

Most commonly due to chronic bronchitis. This disease is essentially due to irritants such as industrial or tobacco smoke inhaled over long periods of time. The result is bronchial damage and constant excessive production of sputum punctuated by frequent infection (exacerbation) especially during winter months.

Antibiotics (see p.108)
The most common infecting organisms are H. influenzae and the pneumococcus. Tetracycline, (p.122) ampicillin (p.115) and co-trimoxazole (p.123) are commonly used both in treatment and in prophylaxis.

Bronchodilators
In acute exacerbations some reactive bronchoconstriction may respond to β-stimulants such as Salbutamol and theophyllinates (e.g. choline theophyllinate). Physiotherapy and cessation of smoking are essential adjuncts to treatment. Corticosteroids are anti-inflammatory; in addition to relaxing bronchial smooth muscle they also reduce mucosal swelling during acute exacerbations.

Mucolytics
Several agents are available for thinning tenacious sputum in the hope of improving expectoration and ventilation. None are of proved value and water vapour inhalations are at least as effective and considerably cheaper.

OXYGEN

Oxygen in lung disease is as important as any of the above drugs and if misused can be equally dangerous.

Acute respiratory/ventilatory disturbances

Acute disease states such as pneumonia, left ventricular failure, pneumothorax, and acute asthma are all characterized by anoxia and reflex hyperventilation. The blood CO_2 level commonly falls and oxygen may be administered to advantage in high concentration.

Chronic obstructive airways disease

The situation is quite different. Chronically raised levels of CO_2 in the blood are tolerated over a period of time and fail to stimulate ventilation. The only stimulus to ventilation which remains is hypoxaemia. If this stimulus is removed by the inappropriate use of high concentrations of oxygen, ventilation may fall resulting in further retention of CO_2; coma and death due to hypercapnia may ensue.

Administration

In the dental situation oxygen may be needed in the acute asthmatic attack (p.198), or in anaphylactic shock (p.195). In either case cyanosis is liable to develop as evidence of hypoxia. Most frequently, of course, oxygen is delivered as a gas-oxygen mixture during general anaesthesia. As a rule **No patient with obstructive airways disease should receive more than 28% oxygen** (Room air = 21%).

Methods of Administration
Pure oxygen may be administered in an emergency by the following means.
1   Ambu-bag and rubber mask: This piece of equipment should be standard in the dental surgery in order to meet emergency situations such as those outlined above. By applying pressure, the soft rubber rim of the mask can be made to fit perfectly over the face; by attaching an oxygen line to the bellows, 100 % oxygen can be supplied under intermittent positive pressure.
2   Anaesthetic machine: the machine has the facility to supply oxygen of any chosen concentration under positive pressure through the Ambu face mask.
3   Closed mask: Up to 80 % inspired oxygen may be achieved with a plastic M.C. mask or similar. The patient expires through perforations in the mask.
     For patients with obstructive airways disease the following may be used to limit the concentration of inspired oxygen:
1   Anaesthetic machine, adjusted to supply 28 % oxygen-air mixture.
2   'Venti-Mask' — a plastic mask which operates on the Venturi principle by directing a jet of oxygen across an aperture in the mask open to room air. The force of the jet determines the final concentration of oxygen in the inspired air. 'Venti-masks' designed to give various fixed concentrations of oxygen are available.

Side-effects

Respiratory depression
Risk to patients with obstructive airways.

Pulmonary atelectasis
The alveoli of the anaesthetised patient may be filled predominantly with oxygen which is a soluble gas. Obstruction to bronchioles caused by tenacious mucus or rarely inadvertently inhaled oral debris may result in collapse of the segment distal to the obstruction. Minor atelectasis is not uncommon in heavy smokers or chronic bronchitics following general anaesthesia.

COUGH

Coughing is a usually protective reflex which results from irritation to the mucosa of the airways. It is most commonly due to excessive secretions but the causes are protean. Drugs which encourage coughing include expectorants and mucolytics; those which suppress it are termed cough suppressants.

Expectorants

The majority act on the stomach — a secondary reflex stimulates coughing and may thin out viscous bronchial secretions. A vast number of proprietary expectorant mixtures are available; their principal ingredients are iodides, squill (sea-onion plant), ipecacuanha ('Brazil root') and quiacols. Most have not been subjected to clinical trial but are harmless and apparently effective remedies. Mild sedatives of the antihistamine (phenothiazine) group are commonly added.

Cough Suppressants

Peripheral action
Pharyngeal irritation may respond to demulcents such as liquorice lozenges which coat the mucosa and reduce irritation. A cough linctus, strictly speaking, is a simple demulcent.

Central action
Opiates (p.145) have a cough-suppressant action on the medullary centre of the brain stem. Where indicated, i.e. terminal bronchial carcinoma — morphine or methadone (longer acting, less narcotic) are effective and valuable drugs.

The non-addictive members are safe and effective suppressants in more trivial situations, e.g. codeine phosphate.

EPHEDRINE DECONGESTANTS

Action
Releases stored noradrenaline from nerve terminals. In its context as a decongestant it causes vasoconstriction of mucosal arterioles, reducing oedema and mucosal secretions. It is usually applied as nasal drops.

Toxicity
If given orally, the absorbed dose has a stimulant action on the CNS giving rise to alertness, anxiety and insomnia limiting its usefulness by this route. Nasal drops are not absorbed sufficiently to cause this problem.

RESPIRATORY STIMULANTS (analeptics)

All analeptic drugs are general CNS stimulants and are liable to cause convulsion. They may have limited value in states of hypoventilation, such as hypercapnic coma (due for instance to the misapplication of oxygen) but should always be considered a secondary measure. Clearing of the airways and assisted ventilation are far more important. (A controlled trial in which nikethamide was used in severe barbiturate poisoning showed a significantly greater death rate among the nikethamide group.)

4.6   DYSRHYTHMIAS OF THE HEART

1   Drugs used principally in atrial dysrhythmias
Digoxin
β-adrenoceptor blockers
   Propranolol
   Oxprenolol

2   Drugs used principally in ventricular dysrhythmias
Procainamide
Lignocaine
Phenytoin
Mexilitene

3   Atropine

PHYSIOLOGY

The right and left sides of the heart, although functionally separate, share the same conduction system and beat synchronously.

The atria contract while the ventricles are at rest (diastole) followed by contraction of the ventricles while the atria rest (systole). For maximum efficiency the timing of this sequence (known as the cardiac cycle) is critical.

Dysrhythmias are the result of distrubances in the sequence of electrical activity and treatment is aimed at restoring it to normal.

Physiologically, cardiac tissue differs from skeletal muscle in three major respects:

1. Inherent rhythmicity (automaticity)
Isolated pieces of cardiac tissue will depolarize regularly and spontaneously in the absence of an external stimulus.

Should a block occur in the conducting system of the intact heart the tissues distal to it will assume the frequency of discharge of the tissue just beyond the block.

Two facts of therapeutic importance arise:
(a)   Ventricular contraction does not depend upon absolute integrity of the conducting system; it will continue to occur, though at a much slower rate, despite total interruption of the atrio-ventricular node.
(b)   Suppression of the conduction system positively encourages automaticity of heart muscle by releasing it from the influence of the primary pacemaker's impulses.

Dysrhythmias may arise in two ways: disease (usually ischaemia) may block the conduction system (heart block), or stimulate secondary (autonomous) pacemaker activity of a frequency sufficient to over-ride the sinoatrial node (ecopic tachycardia). Drugs may do both simultaneously.

2. Duration of action potential
The action potential of cardiac tissue lasts considerably longer than that of skeletal muscle or nerve, and during this time the tissue is entirely refractory to further stimulation. The duration of this refractory period thus limits the frequency at which the tissue can discharge. Drugs can significantly alter the refractory period.

3. High sensitivity to transmitters such as adrenaline and acetylcholine
Adrenaline is the chemical transmitter of sympathetic (adrenergic) nerves and also circulates freely in the blood stream; acetylcholine is the transmitter of parasympathetic (cholinergic) nerves. The heart is highly sensitive to both transmitters.

Adrenergic stimulation

Sympathetic nerves innervate principally pacemaking and conducting tissues. All areas of the heart respond to circulating adrenaline. Adrenergic stimulation reduces the refractory period and the heart rate accordingly rises. Adrenaline may also cause instability of the membrane potential of pacemaker or myocardial cells; resultant oscillations may trigger random depolarizations throughout the heart (ectopic beats). Palpitations are familiar following a sudden fright.

Cholinergic stimulation

The vagus nerve innervates mainly the nodal (sinoatrial and atrioventricular) tissues. Vagal stimulation increases the refractory period of conducting tissue and will reduce the heart rate by reducing pacemaker frequency.

Electrolytes
A fall in serum potassium concentration shortens the refractory period and an increase can cause loss of spontaneous activity owing to permanent depolarization, resulting in cardiac standstill (arrest).

DRUGS USED TO TREAT DYSRHYTHMIAS

Drugs act in one of two ways:
1 Directly, either by altering the refractory period or by influencing excitability and automaticity. The response of the intact heart to anti-dysrhythmic drugs is often complex because nervous and hormonal reflexes always influence the result. In addition, many commonly used drugs exert cardiac side-effects (e.g. antidepressants, anaesthetics) and some may alter serum electrolytes (thiazide diuretics, carbenoxolone).
2 Indirectly, by amplifying or blocking the effects of natural transmitters, thereby altering the refractory periods of cardiac tissue.

DIGOXIN

Digoxin has two therapeutically important actions in the treatment of dysrhythmias:
1 Vagal action.
2 It lengthens the refractory period of conducting tissue (but shortens that of muscle).
   Accordingly digoxin is used to treat fast atrial dysrythmias. It has no slowing effect on the atrial muscle but blocks conduction of a proportion of atrial impulses to the ventricles thereby reducing the ventricular rate.

Toxicity
The elderly are relatively intolerant to digoxin. Toxicity may result from excessive plasma concentrations (commonly overdosage, renal failure) or from *low serum potassium levels* (hypokalaemia) which potentiate the action of digoxin on heart muscle. The specific effects are:

1   *Heart block.* Excessive depression of the A-V node may so lengthen its refractory period as to prevent transmission of all atrial impulses. The result is complete heart block and the ventricles beat independently and slowly (24-40/min).

2   *Automaticity.* Over-digitalized muscle fibres fail to respond to propagated impulses (i.e. become non-excitable) but simultaneously develop spontaneous and autonomous activity. The characteristic picture with progressive digoxin toxicity is bigeminy (propagated ventricular impulse alternating with autonomous ventricular discharges) lapsing into atrial tachycardia with atrio-ventricular block. Further toxicity leads to ventricular flutter and fibrillation.

Kinetics
(See section on heart failure). Digoxin is a kidney-dependent drug.

β-ADRENOCEPTOR BLOCKING DRUGS

Those tissue receptors sensitive to sympathetic stimulation may be of the a or β (β_1 or β_2) type. Cardiac adrenoceptors are all of the β_1 type and the effects of sympathetic stimulation of the heart (neural or humoral) have been discussed above.

The effects of β-blockade

Advantage
· Reduction in heart rate.
· Conversion of atrial tachycardias to normal sinus rhythm.
· Suppression of automaticity.

Unlike digoxin (p.77) β-blocking drugs have a primary effect on the cardiac pacemaker. By prolonging the refractory period of the sino-atrial node, sinus tachycardia may be slowed. Stabilization of the resting potential may abolish ectopic premature beats (palpitations) which are common in situations of high adrenergic activity such as emotional or physical stress.

Disadvantage
Lack of organ specificity. The early β-blocking drugs such as propranolol lack specificity, tending to block β_2 as well as β_1 adrenoceptors. The

effects of non-selective blockade are:
· bronchospasm in those predisposed (bronchitis, asthma);
· suppression of the physical signs of high adrenergic activity;
· inability to convert glycogen rapidly to glucose.

The clinical side-effects of indiscriminate β-blockade are acute asthmatic attacks in the predisposed, lack of early signs of hypoglycaemia in the diabetic (all the signs except coma are due to the reflex adrenaline response to a falling blood sugar) and the inability of the diabetic to produce sugar rapidly from stored glycogen in times of need.

Quinidine-like effects (suppression of conducting and myocardial tissue). The danger lies in the use (or rather misuse) of β-blockade in heart failure. The failing heart *depends* on intense sympathetic drive and the combined effect of β-blockade and direct myocardial suppression can only lead to further deterioration in cardiac performance.

Drugs available

A number of β-adrenoceptor blocking drugs are available. The two most widely used are:
Propranolol. Can be considered the 'parent' drug. Potent, but it has the disadvantages noted above.
Oxprenolol. Considered to cause less cardiac depression.

Kinetics
All are well absorbed orally and are metabolized by the liver.

β-blockade and anaesthesia: Propranolol modifies the body's reaction to stress and should ideally be withdrawn 24 hours before surgery using general anaesthesia. In emergency situations, general anaesthesia may be used in the presence of propranolol provided that:
· Unbalanced vagal tone is blocked by atropine to prevent bradycardia and hypotension.
· Anaesthetics associated with myocardial depression (ether, chloroform, cyclopropane, trichloroethylene) are avoided.

OTHER DRUGS FOR DYSRHYTHMIA TREATMENT

Procainamide

Procainamide is derived from the local anaesthetic procaine by simple substitution of an amide for an ester linkage (this confers upon procainamide a much longer duraton of action and fewer CNS effects). Local anaesthetic effect and quinidine-like effects are synonymous terms, and the actions of

procainamide on the heart are essentially similar to those of quinidine:
Prolongation of atrial refractory period.
Reduced excitability in all tissues (elevation of the threshold potential).
Suppression of spontaneous pacemaker activity.

Toxicity
Hypersensitivity reaction (fever, arthralgia, histamine mediated skin
eruptions).
Agranulocytosis. Rare.
Syndrome resembling SLE (systemic lupus erythematosis) on chronic
usage.

Lignocaine

A local anaesthetic familiar to dentists. It differs from procainamide and
quinidine in a number of important respects:
· Very rapid onset and offset of action, permitting greater flexibility of
use.
· Causes little change in the atrio-ventricular conduction time.
· Greater tendency to cause convulsions.
· Cannot be administered orally (owing to brief duration of action).
· Fundamentally different structure; a safe alternative in cases of procaina-
mide hypersensitivity.
  Note: Mexilitene was introduced during 1976 as an alternative to
lignocaine and long-term procainamide.

Phenytoin

Nowadays considered the drug of choice in major epilepsy, it also has
important (and unique) actions on the heart. Phenytoin is used only in the
acute treatment of dysrhythmias and is the drug of choice in digoxin
poisoning of the heart.

Atropine

Atropine blocks vagal stimulation of the heart by competitive antagonism
of acetylcholine. The important effects are:
1 Increase in heart rate
2 Improvement in atrio-ventricular conduction; the refractory period is
reduced.

4.7   ORAL ULCERATION

Antibacterial	Metronidazole Neomycin Penicillin Tetracycline
Antiviral	Idoxuridine
Antifungal	Amphotericin Nystatin
Protective Covering	Carboxymethyl cellulose
Antiseptics	Chlorhexidine Hydrogen peroxide Sodium perborate Sodium hypochlorite
Local analgesic	Choline salicylate paste
Locally applied steroids	Hydrocortisone Triamcinalone
Liquorice derivative	Carbenoxolone
Hormones	Oestrogen
Caustic agents	Copper sulphate Phenol Silver nitrate

An ulcer is a break in surface continuity of skin or mucous membrane and the causes may be:
· Traumatic
· Infective
· Systemic
  Neoplastic
· Drug-induced
· Unknown (Aphthous − herpetiform ulcers)
   Where a cause can be established treatment is specific, otherwise it is symptomatic.

TRAUMA

The commonest form of oral ulceration. It may be chemical, e.g. aspirin burn or mechanical, e.g. due to a rough filling, denture, broken tooth etc. The cause must be removed. Meanwhile the ulcer may be coated with a protective covering of carboxymethyl cellulose paste which adheres to the moist mucous membrane.

Sodium carboxymethyl cellulose paste: smear over the ulcer as required.

INFECTIVE:

Bacterial

Acute ulcerative gingivitis
There is an association with the spirochaete Borrelia vincenti and Bacillus fusiformis, but poor oral hygiene and smoking are predisposing factors. Mouthwashes of hydrogen peroxide and sodium perborate are effective in debridement owing to their effervescent action. The organisms are sensitive to (systemic) penicillin, but metronidazole is increasingly used and is particularly useful in cases of penicillin hypersensitivity. (p.113).
· Hydrogen peroxide solution BP (20 vol. strength)
Dilute 1 part in 4 parts water
· Sodium perborate mouthwash, buffered
Dissolve sachet in a tumbler of water.
· Phenoxymethyl penicillin tablets 250 mg q.i.d.
· Metronidazole tablets 200 mg b.d. on the first day, then 200 mg t.i.d. for two more days.

Tuberculosis
May first present as a chronic ulcer of the mucous membrane secondary to pulmonary tuberculosis. The ulcer will heal after institution of systemic antituberculous therapy.

Syphilis
All three classical stages of syphilis may produce oral ulcers — primary chancre of lip or tongue; snail track ulcers of the mucous membrane in the seconday stage; gumma causing deep palatal perforations in tertiary syphilis.
    Treatment (parenteral penicillin) is the province of the medical practitioner or venereologist.

Viral

Primary herpes
Caused by *Herpesvirus hominis*. Primary herpetic stomatitis is seen mainly

in children but increasingly in young adults. A tetracycline mouthbath reduces symptoms probably by countering secondary infection. The specific anti-viral agent Idoxuridine may be useful either painted on the lesion with a sterile brush or cotton wool pledget or taken as a mouthbath.

· Tetracycline mixture 2%
Hold in the mouth for 2-3 minutes. Repeat t.i.d. for 2-3 days.
· Idoxuridine Paint 0.1%
Paint: apply the solution to the ulcer q.i.d. for 2-3 days.
Mouthbath: hold in the mouth for 2-3 minutes. Repeat t.i.d. for 2-3 days.

Recurrent herpes
The familiar cold sore. Idoxuridine paint may prevent replication of the virus and appears effective in practice. Alternatively a hydrocortisone cream combined with an antibiotic like neomycin to prevent secondary infection may be tried. The cream must be applied at the prodromal stage. It has no effect on an established lesion.
· Hydrocortisone cream 1%
· Neomycin cream 0.5 g.

Herpes zoster and chickenpox
Caused by the same virus. Zoster is distinguished by its unilateral and anatomical distribution. The ulcers are more painful than Herpes simplex. Symptomatic treatment, e.g. with a tetracycline mouthbath is indicated.

Infectious mononucleosis
Caused by a Herpes virus. Oral ulceration may be a feature. Treatment is symptomatic.

Herpangina and hand, foot and mouth disease
These are transient conditions caused by an A-type Coxsackie virus and treatment (if any) is symptomatic.

Fungal

Moniliasis: Denture sore mouth is the commonest form and produces a red haemorrhagic ulcer. The cause is secondary infection by candida of palatal tissue traumatized by a poorly-fitting denture. Besides anti-fungal treatment with Nystatin or Amphotericin (p.125) a new denture should be made and denture hygiene improved, e.g. by immersing the denture overnight in an antiseptic solution.
· Amphotericin Lozenges 10 mg q.i.d.
Mixture 100 mg in 1 ml as mouthbath q.i.d. may be usefully swallowed.
Ointment 3% smeared on the dentures fitting surface.

· Nystatin Tablets 500,000 units q.i.d. allow to dissolve slowly in mouth. Mixture 100,000 units in 1 ml as a mouth bath q.i.d. no value in swallowing as the action is purely local. Ointment 100,000 units applied to the denture.
· Disinfectant for denture. Sodium hypochlorite 1%.

SYSTEMIC DISEASE

In deficiency conditions treatment is by appropriate replacement therapy. Symptomatic relief can be obtained by using a covering agent, a tetracycline mouthbath or topically-applied steroids.

Blood disorders

Anaemia
Glossitis and oral ulceration are features of all the anaemias. Diagnosis includes blood examination with treatment by replacement therapy (see p.63).

Agranulocytosis
A condition in which circulating polymorphs are greatly reduced. It may be idiopathic or secondary to irradiation, aplastic anaemia, leukaemia. Agranulocytosis may also result from idiosyncracy to drugs such as phenylbutazone, chloramphenicol, sulphonamides, carbimazole. Treatment is by replacement of white cells. The oral condition improves markedly when oral hygiene is improved. Hydrogen peroxide and Sodium perborate mouthwashes are indicated.

Leukaemias
Characterized by an uncontrolled excess of functionless white blood cells. Oral symptoms occur in 20 % of cases, the presence of local irritants being the precipitating factor. Severe ulceration may follow minor trauma of the oral mucosa.
Mouthwashes as for agranulocytosis. A carboxymethyl covering paste may help to protect the denuded mucosa.

Skin conditions

Lichen planus, lupus erythematosis, pemphigus vulgaris, pemphigoid
Inflammatory conditions of unknown aetiology often presenting with painful oral ulceration. The use of topically-applied steroids is justified. Intermittent topical applications are not absorbed significantly although

sustained administration may cause suppression of the hypothalamic – pituitary-adrenal axis (p.156). Severe cases may require hospital admission and systemic steroid therapy.

· Hydrocortisone lozenges 2.5 mg b.d., t.i.d. or q.i.d.
one lozenge is dissolved slowly next to the ulcer.

· Triamcinolone 0.1% in carboxymethyl cellulose paste
apply directly to the lesion with an orange stick or plastic instrument q.i.d.
(The paste is mechanically protective enabling the corticosteroid to act for a longer period.)

Erythema multiforme
May be a manifestation of drug hypersensitivity e.g. to sulphonamides, penicillin or barbiturates. The condition has been known to follow infection by herpes simplex and deep x-ray therapy.
Treatment: The widespread bleeding erosions may be treated with topical steroids. Severe cases may require admission for systemic steroid therapy.
Note: Related syndromes: Beçet, Reiter, Stevens-Johnson.

Gastro-intestinal conditions

Crohn's Disease
A granulomatous condition of unknown aetiology. Oral ulceration may be a presenting factor. The overall management is a medical/surgical problem.
Treatment: topical steroids.

NEOPLASTIC

Squamous cell carcinoma comprises 95 % of all oral malignancies. It often presents as an indurated ulcer.
Treatment: Excision or Radiotherapy.
If any ulcer persists for two or three weeks a blood examination should be made and, if negative, a biopsy.

DRUG INDUCED

1   Secondary to agranulocytosis caused by a drug which has depressed the bone marrow (p.64).
2   Following prolonged exposure to heavy metals (e.g. bismuth, lead, mercury) or to gold.
3   Fixed drug eruption. A localized hypersensitivity to certain drugs (e.g. barbiturates, salicylates, tetracyclines) presenting as a mouth ulcer.
4   Erythema multiforme.

UNKNOWN

Aphthous and Herpetiform Ulcers

Recurrent painful ulcers of the oral mucosa. Although the aetiology is unknown there may be an auto-immune mechanism. Symptomatic relief is the aim of treatment, at first with simple remedies. Steroids are a last resort.
Protective paste. Carboxymethyl cellulose gel.

Analgesic. Choline salicylate paste 8 % apply directly to the lesion q.i.d.
     Contra-indication: aspirin allergy.

Antiseptic mouthwash. Phenol and Alkaline Mouthwash (phenol 3% potassium hydroxide 3 %) dilute 10 ml in 100 ml warm water.
     Chlorhexidine 2 % (dilute with an equal volume of water).

Antibiotic. Tetracycline mouthbath 2 %.

Topical steroids to suppress the inflammatory reaction. Hydrocortisone lozenge 2.5 mg Triamcinalone 0.1 % in carboxymethyl cellulose paste.

Liquorice derivative. Carbenoxolone sodium gel 2 % smear the gel over the affected area. Repeat q.i.d. until the symptoms abate.

Oestrogen therapy
Aphthous ulceration may occur premenstrually and improvement may follow taking the contraceptive pill.

Caustic agents
Destroy the nerve endings, but cause tissue damage which delays healing. The medicament is applied directly to the ulcer.
Phenol.
Silver Nitrate.
Copper Sulphate.

4.8   ADVERSE ORAL DRUG REACTIONS

The following adverse drug reactions may present to the dentist:
Skin
Urticaria: Allergy, e.g. to penicillin.
Oedema lip: Angio-neurotic oedema — hypersensitivity, e.g. to pencillin, aspirin.

Jaundice: Liver damage or obstruction due to halothane, chlorpromazine.

Gingivae
Hyperplasia: Phenytoin. Barbiturates. Oral contraceptive.
Pigmentation: Heavy metals, phenindione.

Tongue
Black stain: Iron preparations.

Stomatitis
Oral ulceration: Drugs causing agranulocytosis.
Stevens-Johnson: Sulphonamide, phenobarbitone.
Erythematous area: Fixed drug reaction, e.g. due to phenolphthalein, barbiturates, meprobamate.
Lichenoid eruption: Keratosis caused by chlorpropamide, chlorothiazide, heavy metals.
Xerostomia: Atropine, antihistamines, tricyclic antidepressants, barbiturates.

Teeth
Rampant caries: May follow xerostomia.
Staining: Tetracycline.
Fluorosis: Fluoride in excess of 2 ppm.

4.9   GASTRO-INTESTINAL DISORDERS

Peptic ulcer	Cimetidine
	Sodium bicarbonate
	Magnesium hydroxide
	Magnesium trisilicate
	Aluminium hydroxide
	Propantheline
	Carbenoxolone sodium
Vomiting	Promethazine
	Cyclizine
	Chlorpromazine
	Metoclopramide
Diarrhoea	Codeine phosphate
	Diphenoxylate
	Propantheline
	Kaolin

Constipation   Bisacodyl
                                  Senna
                                  Cascara
                                  Magnesium sulphate
                                  Psyllium seeds
                                  Methylcellulose
                                  Liquid paraffin
                                · Enemeta

The majority of gastro-intestinal disorders are short-lived functional upsets such as vomiting, dyspepsia, constipation, and diarrhoea. As a result, much of the treatment is symptomatic, aimed at tiding the patient over the period of upset. Chronic peptic ulceration is of considerable medical (and economic) importance and lack of natural teeth is a potential factor in its development.

PEPTIC ULCER

The gastro-duodenal mucosa is protected from gastric acid by a layer of mucin. Acid dyspepsia, whether or not accompanied by frank mucosal ulceration, results either from over-production of acid (commonly the case in duodenal ulcer) or from mucin deficiency (thought to be the case in gastric ulceration since acid secretion is usually less than normal). Heartburn is due to reflux of gastric contents which cause spasm of oesophageal muscle and sometimes mucosal ulceration.

Drugs are aimed at restoring the acid-mucin balance by improving the quality of mucin (e.g. carbenoxolone) or by neutralizing gastric acid. There have been recently introduced drugs such as Cimetidine which block the gastric histamine (H_2) receptors which form the final common pathway of all factors which stimulate acid secretion.

Antacids

Action
All are alkaline salts. Their action is entirely symptomatic; they do not promote healing.

Compared to sodium bicarbonate, such salts as magnesium trisilicate and aluminium hydroxide have poor neutralizing power and yet prove successful in practice. They probably offer a demulcent protection to the mucosa, reinforcing the action of mucin.

Kinetics
Sodium salts are readily absorbed. The salts of aluminium, magnesium and calcium are not absorbed.

Toxicity
Sodium bicarbonate, being absorbed, may cause metabolic alkalosis. If taken over long periods with large amounts of milk (a common addiction in ulcer patients) calcium salts may be precipitated and damage the kidney – "milk alkali syndrome".
Magnesium salts cause diarrhoea.

Anti-cholinergic drugs (e.g. propantheline)

Action
Blockade of the vagus nerve which carries parasympathetic impulses to the secretory cell mass of the stomach. They also block other parasympathetic functions and delay gastric emptying which may improve the effectiveness of antacids if taken together. They have no ulcer healing activity.

Liquorice derivatives

The liquorice root is an ancient remedy for oral ulceration. Modern derivatives have been shown to hasten the *healing* of gastric ulcers.

Carbenoxolone Sodium

Action
Liquorice derivative which probably improves quantity and quality of mucin.

Toxicity
It has an aldosterone-like action which may cause sodium retention, hypokalaemia, oedema and hypertension. Carbenoxolone-induced potassium loss may lead to digitalis intolerance and toxicity (p.78).

VOMITING (Emesis)

Vomiting results from stimulation of the emetic centre located in the brainstem. Impulses may arise from
· The cerebral cortex (fear, disgust)
· Gut (disease, irritation, allergy)
· The brainstem chemoreceptor trigger zone (CTZ)

Anti-emetic drugs may act at any of these sites:
Emetic centre: atropine, hyoscine, some classes of antihistamine
Cerebral cortex: sedatives, tranquillizers
Gut: Metoclopromide
CTZ: Chlorpromazine, metoclopromide.
The action of those drugs which act on the emetic centre is related to their anti-cholinergic activity.

Anti-Histamine Group

The anti-histamines are generally taken to include a group of interrelated drugs which have anti-cholinergic activity and block the action of histamine by competitive antagonism of H_1 receptors. Their particular value in vomiting lies in their effect on motion sickness.

Metoclopramide

Action
As an anti-emetic, its principle action is on the brainstem vomiting centre. In addition, metoclopramide relaxes the pyloric sphincter and accelerates gastric emptying.

Toxicity
Extrapyramidal effects manifested by dystonic reactions, lip smacking, etc., are uncommon but respond to anti-cholinergic drugs (hyoscine, atropine) if it is essential to continue the metoclopromide.

Chlorpromazine

This drug is discussed elsewhere (p.169).

DRUGS AS A CAUSE OF VOMITING

Many drugs cause gastric intolerance, rather fewer frank vomiting. The vomiting may result from gastric irritation or from cerebral stimulation (chemoreceptor trigger zone). In the first case (e.g. oral iron preparations) the patient often volunteers the association. The diagnosis of centrally mediated vomiting demands a constant awareness of the possibility by the practitioner. Digoxin is a common cause but a wide variety of drugs may be responsible.

DIARRHOEA

Diarrhoea is due to hypermotility of the colon. This may result from irritation of the wall by infection, drugs or sterile inflammation, or it may have an emotional (psychosomatic) basis.
The result of chronic or severe diarrhoea (i.e. dysentery, ulcerative colitis) is fluid and electrolyte loss.
The cause must be sought; it is not uncommonly due to drugs. Short of treating the cause, drugs are used in treatment for their symptomatic effect.

Diarrhoea due to drugs

Drugs appear to cause diarrhoea in three ways
1   By chemical irritation, e.g. ferrous sulphate, colchicine.
2   By altering the normal bowel flora — antibiotics such as ampicillin and tetracycline.
3   By a pharmacological effect, e.g. purgative drugs.

Drug treatment of diarrhoea

Ideally the underlying cause should be treated (e.g. antimicrobial drugs in some types of dysentery, corticosteroids in acute ulcerative colitis). Symptomatic treatment aims at solidifying the stool either by delaying its passage through the colon to allow maximal reabsorption of water and electrolytes, or by *ad*sorbing the fluid with an inert powder. Specific and symptomatic treatment may be combined to advantage; only symptomatic treatment is considered here:

Drugs which reduce colonic motility
1   Opiate drugs (p.145). Generally they act directly on smooth muscle of the colon maintaining high tone whilst reducing peristalsis. Opiate tinctures may usefully be added to adsorbent powders. Spasm may lead to painful colic.
2   Anti-cholinergic drugs (p.104). Spasmolytic drugs such as propantheline relax smooth muscle and like the opiates, reduce peristalsis.

Adsorbent powders
Kaolin powder is used empirically in diarrhoea and its mode of action is uncertain. It is inert pharmacologically, non-absorbed and therefore safe. Morphine may be added.

CONSTIPATION

Because bowel habit is so variable, constipation is difficult to define. Constipation is better considered in terms of faecal hardness than of frequency of defaecation. Drugs such as codeine and other opiate derivitives may produce constipation and should always be considered as a cause.

DRUGS USED TO TREAT CONSTIPATION (PURGATIVES)

The aim is bowel evacuation. Cathartic or stimulant drugs irritate the bowel into contraction. They often cause discomfort and colic and are positively dangerous if obstruction is present. Laxative drugs either provide bulk for the bowel or soften hardened or impacted faeces; subsequent evacuation is physiological.

Stimulant purgatives (Cathartics)

There are three clinically important sub-groups. All increase motor activity of the intestine. The action of the diphenylmethane (bisacodyl) and anthroquinone (senna and cascara) groups is restricted primarily to the colon so that their action is delayed up to six hours after ingestion. Castor oil acts upon the small intestine and has a rapid and profound effect.

Faecal-softening purgatives (laxatives)

Bulk-forming laxatives
There are two sub-groups
1 Inorganic salts which retain water in the bowel lumen by osmotic pressure. They are principally simple salts (e.g. Glauber's, Rochelle, Epsom) have only a mild action and are little absorbed.
2 Hydrophilic colloids, derived from polysaccaride and cellulose. Natural colloids are found in bran, agar, psyllium seeds, figs and prunes (the latter may also have an irritant effect upon the gut). Several synthetic preparations are effective. All are devoid of systemic effects but have on occasion caused intestinal obstruction.

Emollient laxatives
1 Mineral oils. Liquid paraffin is said to lubricate the colon but its more likely action is either to accelerate peristalsis or influence water absorption.
2 Wetting agents such as dioctyl sodium. They reduce the surface tension of bowel fluids.

4.10   INFECTION

Infections are most commonly due to viruses and bacteria. Occasionally fungi may be responsible; infections due to worms and the antihelminthic drugs used to treat them are not considered here.

Anti-microbial agents attack either the organism's cell wall (or membrane) or interfere with its metabolism. Generally speaking the former group kill the organism while the latter prevent its replication and allow the body's immune defences to destroy the (now static) population of organisms by lysis.

DEFINITIONS

1   Antimicrobial agent: a substance which destroys micro-organisms or suppresses their multiplication or growth.

2   Chemotherapeutic agent: Originally applied to substances which suppress an invading organism without harming the patient. A less specific term than antimicrobial agent, it has more recently included agents used in the treatment of cancer (some of which are also basically antimicrobial).

3   Antibiotic: A chemical substance produced by micro-organisms which has the capacity to suppress or kill other micro-organisms.

THE IDEAL ANTIMICROBIAL

1   Bactericidal rather than bacteristatic.
2   Broad rather than narrow spectrum of activity.
3   High therapeutic ratio.
4   Compatibility with other drugs.
5   Non-sensitizing.
6   Activity unaffected by body exudates (e.g. pus) or inflammatory reaction.
7   No tendency to develop resistance.
8   Effective orally.
9   Rapid onset and long duration of action.
10   Water-solubility and stability.
11   Cheap.

Notes

No individual chemotherapeutic agent can be given with complete safety. Some bactericidal drugs may prove to be bacteristatic in certain situations. Development of bacterial resistance has become a major problem, particularly in the hospital environment. The more recent synthetic agents have become increasingly expensive. Pressure of advertising has led to their wide acceptance in situations where cheaper, less sophisticated preparations may be equally effective. The correct choice of antimicrobial demands a degree of selectivity based on informed opinion.

STRUCTURE OF MICRO-ORGANISMS

Bacterial

Microscopic, rigid-walled unicellular organisms which replicate asexually by binary fission. They consist of an inner protoplasm which is surrounded by a lipoprotein cell membrane with or without a cell wall. The osmotic integrity of the cell is maintained by its rigid cell wall.

Fungi

The moulds, yeasts and actinomycetes are Fungi, a subdivision of Thallophyta, one of the four divisions of the plant kingdom. Individual cells possess a thick chitinous cell wall enclosing the protoplasm which contains cytoplasm and nuclei.

Viruses

Of the order of 10^{-3} the size of bacteria. They exist intracellularly following infection. Under the electron microscope each particle has an electron dense core consisting of nucleic acid surrounded by a protein shell. The type of nucleic acid present — RNA or DNA — characterizes the class of virus.

MODE OF ACTION OF ANTIMICROBIAL DRUGS

Antimicrobial drugs act at one of the following sites:
1   Cell-wall: loss of integrity of the cell-wall results in cell rupture owing to release of osmotic pressure. These drugs are bactericidal.
2   Cell-membrane: the membrane is responsible for active transport process vital to the cells metabolism.
3   Nucleic acid content: interference with ribosomal function disrupts the processes of replication, protein synthesis and information transfer within the cell.
4   Intermediary metabolism: interruption of vital metabolic pathways may lead to suppression of growth and such drugs are usually bacteristatic.

RESISTANCE TO ANTIMICROBIAL ACTION

Clinically, resistance is recognized through failure of the drug to have the desired or anticipated effect, although failure to take the drug as prescribed (non-compliance) is a far commoner cause and must be ruled out first. Resistance may be natural, acquired, or transferred.

Natural
However broad the spectrum, no single agent is effective against all bacteria. In some cases bacteria produce enzymes (e.g. penicillinase) which inactivate the drug.

Acquired
Acquired resistance results from the selective growth of bacterial mutants during exposure to an agent to which the species was initially sensitive. This phenomenon emphasizes the importance of applying antimicrobial therapy early on, in adequate dosage and for a sufficient duration in order to prevent the development of such strains.

Transferred
A bacterium may acquire resistance from its environment.

Cross-resistance
Resistance to a particular drug generally reflects resistance to all other chemically related compounds, and this fact obviously dictates the choice of an alternative antibiotic. Occasionally unpredictable cross-resistance occurs between unrelated drugs.

Combination Therapy
Although the administration of two or more drugs may retard the acquisition of resistance, the incorrect use of combination therapy may reduce the overall antimicrobial effect; bacteristatics should not be used in combination with bactericidal drugs which depend upon active cell growth for their effect. Conversely the combination of two bacteristatic drugs may sometimes result in a bactericidal action.

CONTROL OF INFECTION

Infection can be controlled at three levels:
1   Environmental hygiene   )
2   Personal protection   )   preventive control
3   Treatment of established disease

No matter how effective present or future antimicrobial agents may prove to be in treatment, the prevention of infection is always the more important consideration. Apart from reducing suffering, effective prevention minimizes the exposure of a population to potentially toxic drugs and makes sound economic sense — lost working days may be fewer, the burden on professional and diagnostic facilities is reduced and drug costs are cut.

In terms of preventive dentistry an obvious example is the prevention of chronic periodontal disease.

TREATMENT OF INFECTION

General Principles

Most human infections (because most are trivial) will resolve spontaneously. No drug is free of side-effects. These together dictate a philosophy essential to the proper prescribing of antimicrobial drugs. The immune defences of the body, when intact, provide an extremely effective means of preventing, localizing, and curing infective illness.

Nevertheless antibacterial therapy, when specifically indicated and correctly administered, has done more to change the face of disease in the last thirty years than has any other group of drugs. It is mainly because of abuse (often through ignorance) that many organisms have now become completely resistant to a wide selection of such drugs.

In many cases of infection a presumptive diagnosis can be made clinically (e.g streptococcal throat, staphylococcal abscess) but where facilities permit , an attempt should be made to confirm the suspicion by bacteriological means. Culture techniques have an added advantage that drug sensitivity can be assessed but their value should not be overstressed since the situation in the patient is not always reflected in a laboratory culture medium.

CHOICE OF DRUG

The correct choice of drug depends on the answers to a number of simple questions. It does not depend upon fashions or pressures exerted by the pharmaceutical industry.

Causative organism

Some infective syndromes (e.g. cellulitis) may be caused by different pathogens of widely varying sensitivity; bacteriological examination and culture (always desirable) is in these situations essential. Identification of the organism does not preclude the use of an antimicrobial early in an infection: it demands that cultures be set up prior to giving the drug so that if necessary rational changed in treatment can be made in the light of bacteriological findings.

Antibiotic prophylaxis is a necessary exception to the rule; the use of penicillin in the prophylaxis of infective endocarditis (e.g. prior to dental extraction) is based upon sound experience.

Despite accurate identification of the organism, there is often a wide selection of effective agents and the ultimate choice will depend upon other factors.

Severity of infection

Culture and sensitivity tests can do little more than identify drug-organism compatibility. They do not take into account the dynamics of human infection. Severe infection often demands more potent (and usually more toxic) drugs. To this extent the final choice of drug becomes a clinical decision and the bactericidal drug will probably be preferred to the bacteristatic agent. Many antibacterial drugs can be given either by mouth or parenterally. Where the choice exists, higher plasma levels can be achieved more rapidly parenterally, but this consideration is usually only relevant in severe infections and special situations such as the prophylaxis of infective endocarditis (p.117). In simple infections, oral administration is usually preferred.

Therapeutic ratio and potency

The sheer number of antimicrobial drugs now available has to some extent blurred the perspective of choice. With the advent and successful advertising of synthetic penicillins (such as ampicillin and amoxicillin) the natural preparations have lost their pride of place. In specific situations (e.g. streptococcal throat), penicillin V & G are many times more potent than their modern counterparts and are extremely safe. In such penicillin-sensitive infections there is no case for using the newer semi-synthetic preparations which are less potent and usually more expensive. In less certain situations the choice is often between potent, toxic drugs and less powerful but safer preparations; the decision is clinical and should reflect the balance between potency and severity.

Renal function

Most antimicrobials are renal-dependent for excretion and many are nephrotoxic, particularly in the presence of established renal disease (tetracycline, cephaloridine). Equally important are the raised drug plasma levels likely to result from renal insufficiency; some toxic effects are plasma level dependent.

Cost

Often overlooked. In many cases of minor infection the choice of drug is wide and non-critical. In this situation, cost should be considered.

Note
The primary treatment of abscess is by surgical drainage; the use of anti-microbials will tend to attenuate its development and encourage fibrosis.

INDIVIDUAL DRUGS

PENICILLINS (5 GROUPS)

NATURAL PENICILLINS

Clinical indications
Gram + ve cocci, principally
1   All haemolytic streptococcal infections (e.g. cellulitis, pharyngitis).
2   Penicillin-sensitive staphylococcus infections (e.g. abscesses after adequate drainage).
3   Actinomycosis, anthrax, gas gangrene.
4   Syphylis and gonorrhoea, bacterial endocarditis.

Benzylpenicillin (Penicillin G)

Presentation
Injection Vials, 150 mg powder.
Lozenges 0.6 mg; 3 mg.

Administration
By intramuscular or sometimes intravenous injection.
    The intramuscular route is painful. Frequency normally 6-hourly; dosage depends upon type of infection.

Side-effects
1   Allergic skin manifestations, usually in the form of an itchy rash, are the commonest clinical problem and respond to withdrawal of the drug. More serious reactions include generalized urticaria (with or without

pharyngeal oedema) asthma and cardiovascular collapse (anaphylactic shock, p. 194).

2   Glossitis. Care should be taken to avoid treating the glossitis which occasionally accompanies the (rarely justified) use of penicillin lozenges, with yet more penicillin.

Phenoxymethylpenicillin (Penicillin V)

Presentation
Tablets 125 mg, *250 mg*
Capsules 125 mg, *250 mg*
Elixir 62.5 mg, 125 mg, 250 mg in 5 ml
Mixture 62.5 mg, 125 mg, 250 mg in 5 ml

Administration
The usual adult dose is 250 mg q.i.d.
Elixir and mixture are for use in children:
>   Up to 1 year   62.5 mg q.i.d
>   1-5 year   125 mg q.i.d
>   6-12 year   250 mg q.i.d.

Both should be stored in a cool place and used within one week of preparation.

Side-effects
Allergy is the major problem and a history of past reactions should always be sought. Diarrhoea may occur.

PENICILLINASE – RESISTANT PENICILLINS

Clinical indications: Penicillinase-producing staphylococcal infections (abscesses, wound-infections etc.)

Methicillin

Presentation
Injection Vials, 1 g powder.

Administration
Intramuscular injection, 1-2 g t.i.d or q.i.d (adults).
Following preparation the solution should be stored between 2° -10° C and used within two days.

Side-effects
Allergic manifestations similar to other penicillins. Superinfection following prolonged use.

Cloxacillin

Presentation
Injection Vials 250 mg, 500 mg powder.
Capsules 250 mg, 500 mg
Elixir 125 mg in 5 ml.

Administration
By intramuscular injection:
Adults 500 mg − 1 g t.i.d or q.i.d (may be exceeded in certain circumstances).
Children:

Up to 1 year	62.5 mg q.i.d (by aliquot)
1-5 year	125 mg q.i.d ”
6-12 year	250 mg q.i.d ”

The solution should be kept cool and preferably used within 24 hours of preparation.
Orally
Capsules (adults)   500 mg − 1 g t.i.d
Elixir (children)
    1-5 years   5-10 ml q.i.d
Gastric absorption is not reliable. The elixir should be stored in a cool place and used within 7 days.

AMPICILLIN

Clinical indications:
1   Sensitive urinary infections
2   Infective exacerbations of chronic bronchitis
3   Septicaemia − in conjunction with cloxacillin
4   Typhoid fever

Presentation
Capsules 250 mg; 500 mg
Tablets (paediatric) 125 mg
Mixture 125 mg in 5 ml
Injection Vials 100 mg; 250 mg; 500 mg powder
(Water for injection supplied).

Administration
The vast majority of prescriptions are for oral ampicillin:
Capsules (adults) 250-500 mg q.i.d

Paed. tablets	)	Up to 1 year	62.5 mg q.i.d
Paed. mixture	)	1-5 year	125 mg q.i.d
Paed. injection	)	6-12 year	250 mg q.i.d
(i.m. or i.v.)			
Injection (adults)			250-750 mg q.i.d

Side-effects
Allergic rash (usually macular) and diarrhoea are the commonest reactions. Ampicillin should be avoided in patients with glandular fever (infectious mononucleosis) and chronic lymphatic leukemia because 90 % of such patients constantly develop a rash. If toxicity arises, the drug should be withdrawn. Rashes may develop up to six weeks following cessation of treatment.
Note: Amoxycillin has recently been introduced with certain minor advantages over ampicillin, but is basically similar.

CARBENICILLIN SODIUM

Clinical indications:
1   Pseudomonas infections
2   Proteus urinary infections resistant to other antimicrobials. Gentamicin displays synergy with carbenicillin and these drugs are commonly administered together; they are generally reserved for pseudomonas infections.

 ## LONG-ACTING PREPARATIONS

Clinical indications: as for benzylpenicillin but excluding situations where high blood levels are essential.

Procaine penicillin

Presentation
Injection Vials 300 mg powder.

Administration
For intramuscular injection only. Provides adequate tissue levels for 24 hours.

Dose adults		300-900 mg daily
Children:	Up to 1 year	150 mg
	1-5 year	300 mg
	6-12 year	600 mg

If kept at room temperature the injection should be used within 24 hours of preparation.

Procaine penicillin Injection, Fortified

Presentation
Vials 300 mg procaine penicillin + 60 mg benzylpenicillin powder.

Triplopen

Benethamine penicillin G 475 mg)
Procaine penicillin 250 mg   )
Sodium penicillin G 200 mg   )
Vials of powder   )
Acts for 2-3 days providing low but sustained penicillin plasma levels.

Allergic reactions may result from the use of all long-acting penicillins but the risk of procaine-induced anaphylaxis must also be remembered.

Long-acting penicillins are often useful in the unreliable patient (who may default on oral preparations) and those in whom treatment is socially essential (e.g. veneral disease).

PROPHYLAXIS AGAINST INFECTIVE ENDOCARDITIS

It is not unknown for a dentist to perform an extraction in total ignorance of his patient's heart disease with the subsequent development of fatal endocarditis. The reason is most frequently a simple failure of communication. Doctor, patient and dentist should all be aware of the significance of congenital heart disease or acquired valve disease in relation to dental surgery. The doctor should routinely inform the appropriate dentist when the lesion is first discovered; the patient should be in a position to volunteer the information; the dentist should always seek to elicit the fact and his is the ultimate responsibility. Such precautions apply not only to dental extraction but to any procedure liable to cause bacteraemia, e.g. scaling, gingivectomy, pulpectomy.

In medical practice the pattern of infective endocarditis has changed over recent years. Non bacterial (viral, coxiella and even fungal) pathogens are becoming increasingly important and the term infective endocarditis is now preferred to SBE (subacute bacterial endocarditis). Urinary tract instrumentation such as cystoscopy and catheterization are now probably commoner precipitants of endocarditis than dental surgery but this in no way exonerates the dentist from exercising careful prophylaxis in those at risk.

The at-risk groups include:
1   *Congenital heart disease* —
Ventricular septal defect
Patent ductus arteriosus
Bicuspid aortic valve
Pulmonary valve stenosis
Coarctation of the aorta
2   *Acquired heart lesions:*
Rheumatic: mitral incompetence; aortic incompetence
Post-surgical: Cardiac surgery is increasingly available even to the most serious cases of congenital or acquired lesions of the heart. The sites of surgical scarring (e.g. anastomosis) or insertion of prostheses, are potentially at risk from infection.

Notes
It should be remembered that oral sepsis is in itself a factor predisposing to infective endocarditis in those with cardiac damage.

Not every patient with a history of rheumatic fever has cardiac damage. A cardiologist's opinion may obviate the need for penicillin which always carries a finite risk of anaphylaxis.

CAUSATIVE ORGANISMS AND PROPHYLAXIS

The dentist risks introducing a transient bacteraemia with organisms of low virulence, principally streptococcus viridans. Accordingly penicillin prophylaxis is indicated and the following regime is commonly employed: Benzylpenicillin (G) 600 mg given i.m. 1 hr preoperatively followed by phenoxymethylpenicillin (V) 500 mg q.i.d. for 2-3 days.

The rationale is to provide high blood levels of penicillin for the period of dental surgery without prior risk of developing resistant organisms. Alternative drugs for those who are penicillin-sensitive or who have recently received penicillin include:
erythromycin (500 mg), or
cephaloridine (500 mg)
given i.m. 1 hr before operation followed by erythromycin or cephalexin 250 mg q.i.d orally for one week as appropriate.

CEPHALOSPORINS

Cephaloridine and Cephalothin

Clinical indications
1   Streptococcal   and   pneumococcal   infections,   in   particular

pneumococcal pneumonia, Strep. pyogenes, throat infection and cellulitis, and Strep. viridans (not faecalis) endocarditis.

2   Staphylococcal infections (excepting those producing large amounts of penicillinase, in the case of cephaloridine).

3   Urinary infection due to E. coli and Proteus mirabilis.

4   Gonorrhoea and early (primary and secondary) syphilis.

Presentation
Cephaloridine. Injection i.m. or i.v.: Vials 250 mg, 500 mg, 1 g powder.
Cephalothin. Injection i.m. or i.v.: Vials 1 g, 4 g (i.v. use).

Administration
By i.m. (painful) or i.v. injection. They are generally used as alternatives in penicillin allergy. (There may, however, be some cross-reactivity between cephalosporins and penicillins).

Side-effects
1   Allergy — mainly skin rash.

2   Nephrotoxicity. The dose should be adjusted to the glomerular filtration rate which must be measured in patients suspected of renal impairment. With high doses of cephaloridine, primary renal damage may occur (particularly in patients taking frusemide).

3   Encephalopathy (twitch, coma) is rare and occurs only with high doses.

4   Their safety in pregnancy is unknown.

Cephalexin

Clinical indications
As for cephaloridine and cephalothin but cephalexin is less potent and has a widely varying effect upon penicillinase-producing Staphylococci.

Presentation
Capsules 250 mg, 500 mg
Tablets 250 mg, 500 mg

Administration
Cephalexin has the advantage of being well absorbed orally. The usual dose is 250-500 mg q.i.d in adults, 25-50 mg/Kg body weight daily for children The dose should be reduced accordingly in renal failure, although cephalexin does not appear to cause kidney damage.

Side-effects
1   Gastro-intestinal upset and diarrhoea.

2   Opportunistic superinfection (e.g. moniliasis; cf tetracyclines).
3   Allergy.

MACROLIDES

Erythromycin

Clinical indications
1   Staphylococcal infections — erythromycin may be useful in extended treatment but offers no advantages over cloxacillin for soft-tissue infection and lincomycin for staphylococcal infection of bone.
2   Infective endocarditis prophylaxis — as an alternative to penicillin.
3   Streptococcal and pneumococcal infections (pneumonia, streptococcal throat, erysipelas, scarlet fever). Erythromycin is the alternative of choice in penicillin-sensitive individuals.
4   Urinary infection.

Presentation
Tablet 250 mg
Chewable tablets 125 mg, 250 mg
Capsules 125 mg, 250 mg
Suspension 125 mg, 250 mg in 5 ml
Drops (paediatric) 100 mg in 1 ml (to be added to a drink).
also available:
Injection i.m. — ampoules 100 mg in 2 ml.

Administration
The usual adult oral dose 500 mg q.i.d, in children 7-10 mg/Kg body weight q.i.d.
Intramuscular injection, 100-200 mg t.i.d, is painful.
Intravenous administration is reserved for severe infections and the dose varies appropriately.
Dosage reduction is not generally necessary in renal disease.

Side-effects
1   Gastro-intestinal upset amounting to nausea, vomiting and diarrhoea is fairly common.
2   Jaundice. Restricted to oral preparations of erythromycin, and often delayed in onset for 10-14 days. It is usually reversible on withdrawal of the drug.

Lincomycin and Clindamycin

Clinical indications
1   Staphylococcal infections. Many consider these to be the drugs of

choice in Staphylococcal osteomyelitis. Both are effective in methicillin (p.114) resistant soft-tissue staphylococcal infection.

2 Streptococcal and pneumococcal infection (tonsilitis, scarlatina, pneumonia, meningitis). Lincomycin or Clindamycin may be satisfactory alternatives in penicillin-sensitive persons.

3 Actinomycosis — both antibiotics have proved successful when given in prolonged courses (i.e. 12 months).

Presentation
Lincomycin. Capsules 250 mg, 500 mg
Paediatric Syrup 250 mg in 5 ml
Injection i.m. or i.v. 600 mg in 2 ml, packaged in a disposable syringe.
Clindamycin. Capsules 75 mg, 150 mg
Paediatric mixture 75 mg in 5 ml.

Administration
The usual adult oral dose for Lincomycin is 500 mg q.i.d, for Clindamycin 150 mg q.i.d. The dose for children should be 10-15 mg/Kg body weight q.i.d of Lincomycin, 15 mg-75 mg q.i.d of clindomycin. The parenteral dosage is similar to the oral and may be doubled in serious infection. I.V. injections should be given slowly. Dosage reduction is necessary in renal failure, and the drugs should be avoided in liver dysfunction.

Side-effects
1 Gastro-intestinal irritation, in particular diarrhoea. The superiority of clindamycin over lincomycin in this respect is contentious.
2 Cardiac arrest has been observed following an intravenous bolus injection of lincomycin.

AMINOGLYCOSIDES

Streptomycin

Clinical indications
1 Tubercolosis — streptomycin is a 'first-line' drug. .
2 Brucellosis.
3 Strep. faecalis endocarditis: Streptomycin + benzylpenicillin in combination.

Side-effects
1 Ataxia and deafness. The risk is related to total dosage and peak levels and it increases with age.
2 Allergy — mainly skin rashes.

TETRACYCLINES

Clinical indications
1   Mouthbath for painful oral ulcerations such as aphthae, lichen planus
and herpetic stomatitis (see also p.98).
2   Surgical infections: reliance upon tetracycline alone is unwise, particularly with hospital-acquired infections where many strains of Staph. aureus
and Gram-negative bacilli are now resistant to tetracycline.
3   Respiratory infection, in particular pneumonia and bronchitis in which
H. influenzae and pneumococcus are common pathogens.
4   Brucellosis. In prolonged infection streptomycin may be added.

Presentation
Tetracycline
    Capsules 100 mg, 250mg
    Tablets 100 mg, 200 mg
    Elixir 125 mg in 5 ml Syrup (paediatric)
    Injection i.m. or i.v. Vials 100 mg, 250 mg.
Chlortetracycline
    Capsules 100 mg, 250 mg
Oxytetracycline
    Capsules 100 mg, 250mg
    Tablets 100 mg (chewable), 250 mg
    Suspension 125 mg in 5 ml (paediatric)
    Injection i.m. Ampoules 100 mg
    i.v. Vials 250 mg
Doxycycline
    Capsules 50 mg, 100 mg
    Suspension 50 mg in 5 ml (paediatric)

Administration
The adult dose of tetracycline, oxytetracycline and chlortetracycline is
250-500 mg q.i.d according to the severity of infection. Children should be
given 5-10 mg/Kg body weight q.i.d.
    It is usual to load doxycycline by giving adults 200 mg the first day and
100-200 mg daily thereafter. The equivalent dose in children is 2.2 mg/Kg
body weight *twice* on the first day and once daily thereafter.
    Tetracycline and oxytetracycline may be given i.m. or i.v. but tissue
irritation is common.
    Tetracyclines in general should be avoided in established renal disease,
although doxycyline is apparently free of nephrotoxicity and does not
accumulate in such patients. Tetracyclines tend to accumulate in advanced
diffuse hepatic disease.
    Chlortetracycline and oxytetracycline are slightly less active than tetra-
cycline against most bacteria but doxycycline is about twice as potent.

Side-effects

1   Discolouration of teeth. The problem is cosmetic and irreversible and will affect both deciduous and permanent dentition according to the period of drug administration. It most frequently follows prolonged or multiple courses of tetracycline and the incidence can be high (20 % of children administered tetracycline in some series).

Yellow staining of the teeth may occur in the following situations:

(a)   Administration to a Mother after the fourth month of pregnancy: the deciduous dentition of the child may be affected.

(b)   Infancy — the deciduous dentition may be affected.

(c)   Childhood; the permanent dentition begins to calcify at six months. The development of anterior crowns is complete by six years so subsequent exposure to tetracycline is unlikely to cause cosmetic disfigurement.

Discolouration is dose-dependent above a critical level. Hypoplasia of the enamel may accompany staining. Doxycycline is said to cause less staining than other tetracyclines.

2   Gastro-intestinal upset. Nausea, dyspepsia and diarrhoea are common. Doxycycline appears to be relatively free of these effects.

3   Superinfection, particularly with Candida albicans (thrush, Monilia).

4   Nephrotoxicity. Deterioration of established renal disease is common during the administration of tetracyclines.

5   Hepatotoxicity. The intravenous use of large doses is dangerous in pregnancy, leading to acute liver failure.

SULPHONAMIDES

All sulphonamides have a similar range of activity but owing to the emergence of resistant organisms, this can no longer be termed broad-spectrum. There are nowadays few specific indications for sulphonamide therapy owing to the availability of better alternatives; the combination of sulphonamide with trimethoprim, however, is a highly effective preparation currently enjoying widespread use.

Trimethoprim and Sulphamethoxazole (Cotrimoxazole)

A highly synergistic and bactericidal combination.

Clinical indications

1   Prophylaxis of meningeal infection in middle-third fractures, particularly if complicated by CSF rhinorrhoea. (Cotrimoxazole diffuses well across the blood-brain barrier).

2   Chronic bronchitis. H. influenzae and the pneumococcus are highly
senstitive.
3   Urinary tract infections.
4   Septicaemia due to Gram-negative bacilli. Although successful, the
current lack of a parenteral preparation of cotrimoxazole limits its application.

Presentation
Tablets Sulphamethoxazole 400 mg, trimethoprim 80 mg.
Paediatric tablets Sulphamethoxazole 100 mg, trimethoprim 20 mg.

Administration
Adults 2 tablets every 12 hr.
Children should be given paediatric tablets, 1 - 4 tablets twice daily accord-
ing to age.

Side-effects
1   Gastric irritation.
2   Bone marrow depression. Pancytopoenia is not uncommon but is
usually mild and reversible upon withdrawal of the drug.
3   Skin rash (1 %).

Sodium fusidate

Clinical indications
Staphylococcal infections, in particular soft tissue infections such as
abscess and furunculosis. It is also indicated in penicillin and methicillin-
resistant staphylococcal septicaemia, osteomyelitis and endocarditis.
(Culture and organism identification are essential because sodium
fisidate is totally ineffective against Gram-negative bacilli).

Presentation
Tablets   250 mg
Suspension, paediatric 35 mg/ml
Injection Vials 500 mg
Ointment   2 %

Administration
Orally the dose is 500 mg t.i.d for adults, up to 15 mg/Kg t.i.d for
children. Parenterally the drug is best given by continuous i.v. infusion,
diluted in isotonic saline; the dose is 500 mg eight-hourly.

Side-effects
Essentially nil.

ANTIFUNGAL ANTIBIOTICS

Nystatin

Clinical indication
Moniliasis (Candida, thrush).

Presentation

Suspension	100 000 IU/ml
Ointment	100 000 IU/g
Tablets	500 000 IU

Administration
Oral moniliasis commonly occurs in debilitated states, in diabetics and in patients on long-term broad-spectrum antibiotic treatment, particularly the tetracyclines. It usually appears as thrush, angular cheilitis or denture stomatitis. Thrush responds to rinsing the mouth with nystatin suspension (5 ml q.id.) or tablets (one q.i.d) which must be allowed to dissolve slowly in the mouth and not swallowed. Angular cheilitis may be treated with the suspension or ointment. Poorly fitting dentures and neglected denture hygiene are predisposing factors to monilial denture stomatitis.

Side-effects
Nausea.

Amphotericin

Clinical indication
1 Topical moniliasis.
2 Systemic fungal infections.

Presentation
Lozenges 10 mg
Suspension 100 mg/ml
Ointment 30 mg/g

Haemophilus—other than meningitis	Pseudomonas	Urine Gram-negative organisms	Proteus spp.	Klebsiella and Coliforms	Esch. Coli	Str. Faecalis	Streptococci and pneumococci	Staph. Aureus—Penicillin resistant	Staph. Aureus—Penicillin sensitive	
							•		•	Penicillin
								•		Flucloxacillin
•		•	•		•	•				Ampicillin/Amoxycillin
	•									Carbenicillin
				•						Cephalosporins
•				•	•					Co-Trimoxazole
•										Tetracycline
	•									Gentamicin
								•		Fusidic Acid

Table 4.1 The major human bacterial pathogens and the first choice in treatment

Administration
May be used as an (often more acceptable) alternative to nystatin in oral moniliasis; one Lozenge q.i.d., dissolved slowly in the mouth or suspension 1 ml q.i.d. as a mouth rinse (must not be diluted prior to use).
Given by injection for systemic fungal infection, amphotericin is highly toxic.

Side-effects
Topical application: nil.
Systemic administration: fever, vomiting, anaemia, renal damage.

ANTIPROTOZOAL DRUGS

Metronidazole

Clinical indications
1   Acute ulcerative gingivitis.
2   Trichomonas infection of the male and female genital tract.

Presentation
Tablets, 200 mg, 400mg.

Administration
Must be regarded as an adjunct to oral hygiene measures.
Metronidazole may be given, 200 mg b.d. on the first day followed by
200 mg t.i.d for two days.

Side-effects
1   Furred tongue and unpleasant taste.
2   Transient rashes.
3   Gastro-intestinal discomfort, occasionally amounting to abdominal
cramps.
4   Tremor, spasticity and ataxia, usually limited to high dosage and
commoner in children.

ANTIVIRAL DRUGS

Idoxuridine

Presentation
Lotion 0.1 %
Ointment 0.5 %.

Clinical indications
Idoxuridine has been most commonly used in dendritic (herpetic) keratitis
of the eye. Herpetic ulceration of oral mucosa and lips may similarly
respond to topical applications. It may be applied by brush or in carboxy-
methylcellulose.

4.11   DISINFECTANTS

Distinction must be made between disinfection and sterilization. Disin-

fection implies that the object is safe to handle but not that it is free of living micro-organisms — as with sterilization. Chemical disinfectants or antiseptics suffer from the following disadvantages:
· Narrow antimicrobial spectrum.
· Inactivated by organic material, e.g. blood, pus, some soaps.
· Unstable solution, chemical becomes inactive and organisms proliferate.

Principles of use
Objects to be disinfected should be clean.
Fresh solutions of disinfectant should be made regularly.
Disinfectant containers must be scrupulously clean.

Uses of disinfectants
Preparation of skin and mucous membrane (value debatable).
Disinfection of objects which cannot be sterilized (e.g. denture).
Disinfection prior to sterilization.
Decontamination of surfaces (from floor boards to bracket table).
Mouthwashes, dentifrices, root canal irrigants.

Comprehensive accounts of disinfectants can be found in any bacteriology text. The accompanying table indicates the range available.

Table 4.2 Disinfectants

Group	Example	Spectrum	Uses	Comments
Phenols	Hycolin, Sudal Para mono Chlorphenol	Wide	Floors Root canal irrigant	Absorbed by rubber
Chloroxylenol	Thymol Dettol	Poor	Thymol mouth wash	Pseudomonas can be cultured in dettol: inactivated by organic matter
Hexachlorophane	Zalpon Cidal soap Phisohex	Gram +ve	soaps, hand creams	Must be used routinely as there is a cumulative antimicrobial effect
Alcohols (70 % strength)	(a) Isopropyl	Wide	Skin	Inactivated by organic matter Expensive
	(b) Ethyl (surgical spirit)		Working Surfaces	
Halogens	Chlorine Hypochlorite	Wide	Bracket table root canal irrigant	Inactivated by organic matter. May corrode metals

Group	Example	Spectrum	Uses	Comments
	Iodine in 70 % alcohol	Wide	Mucous membrane. Rubber dam field	Causes staining. Risk of hypersensitivity. Expensive.
	Povidone Iodine Iodoform		Skin Whitehead's varnish	
Aldehydes	Glutaraldehyde (Cidex)	Wide	Objects unsuitable for sterilizing, e.g. anaesthetic equipment	Expensive
Quaternary Ammonium Compounds	Cetrimide (Cetavlon)	Gram +ve	Detergent	Inactivated by organic matter and soaps. Supports growth of Pseudomonas.
Diguanides	Chlorhexidine (Hibitane) (a) alcoholic	Gram +ve	Skin anaesthetic face mask	Inactiviated by organic matter, soaps, cotton wool, expensive.
	(b) aqueous		(a) Combined with Cetrimide as Savlon for cleaning surfaces & wounds	
			(b) Mouth wash or dental gel	Suppresses bacterial plaque

4.12   ENDOCRINE DISORDERS

Thyroid Disease
Hyperthyroidism
    Propranolol
    Thioureas: Carbimazole, Methylthiouracil, Propylthiouracil
    Potassium perchlorate
    Potassium iodide
Hypothyroidism
    L-thyroxine

Parathyroid Disease
Hypoparathyroidism
    Vitamin D preparations

Adrenal Disease
Hypoadrenalism
   Hydrocortisone (cortisol)
   Fludrocortisone

Ovarian Disease
Ovarian insufficiency
   Oestrogens: Stilboestrol, Ethinyoestradiol
   Progestogens: Norethisterone

Oral Contraceptives
Combined: Oestrogen/progestogen
Sequential: Oestrogen — progestogen
Progestogen alone

Diabetes Mellitus
Insulins
   Short-acting: soluble insulin (crystalline)
   Long-acting: Insulin zinc suspension — semilente, lente, ultralente;
   Protamine zinc insulin; Isophane insulin
Sulphonylureas
   Chlorpropamide
   Tolbutamide
   Glibenclamide
Biguanides
   Phenformin
   Melformin

PATHOPHYSIOLOGY OF ENDOCRINE DISEASE

All healthy endocrine glands function according to demand and are subject to the so-called negative feed-back response. The feed-back pathways are ill-understood and often complex. A gland which continues to secrete irrespective of demand is said to be autonomous and the commonest cause is the growth within the gland of a functioning adenoma. The commonest cause of insufficiency is auto-immune destruction by circulating antibodies and sensitized lymphocytes.

PITUITARY CONTROL

The adrenal gland, thyroid, mammary, ovarian and testicular glands are all under control of pituitary stimulating hormones.

   The pancreatic islet B-cells (insulin) and parathyroid glands are not

under pituitary control but respond to (principally) blood sugar and
calcium levels respectively.

GENERAL PRINCIPLES IN THE CARE OF
ENDOCRINE PATIENTS

1   The treatment and management of endocrine disease require specialist
attention.
2   Replacement therapy should never be withdrawn (even temporarily) or
altered without specialist advice.
3   Dental treatment, particularly any involving anaesthesia should be
carried out in consultation with the medical practitioner and only where
appropriate materials for resuscitation are available (e.g. glucose for
diabetics; hydrocortisone for those with Addison's disease).

APPLICATION OF DRUGS TO ENDOCRINE
DISEASE

Functional disturbance of an endocrine gland may lead to over-activity
(hyperfunction) or insufficiency. In those glands whose function is dependent on pituitary stimulation, over-activity or insufficiency are in many
cases the result of pituitary disease; a pituitary tumour can produce
excess secretion or alternatively cause pressure necrosis leading to pituitary
insufficiency.

SPECIFIC DISORDERS

PITUITARY DISEASE

The pituitary gland has traditionally been termed the conductor of the
endocrine orchestra in reference to its function as a trophic stimulator of
other endocrine glands.
    Pituitary adenomas, whether functional or destructive, are treated by
surgery or radiotherapy. Destructive pituitary lesions are commonly
characterized by an early failure of gonadotrophins and growth hormone,
followed later by loss of adrenocorticotrophic hormone (ACTH) and
thyroid-stimulating hormone (TSH). Replacement therapy is given where
needed according to regular assessment of end-organ (e.g. adrenal, thyroid)
function. Growth hormone replacement is not required after puberty and
gonadotrophins are seldom indicated in the peri- or post-menopausal
female.

Replacement Therapy

1 Gonadotrophin deficiency: Substitution therapy in the female with cyclical oestrogens and progestogens (ovarian hormones) can produce normal menstruation and improve secondary sexual (e.g. breast) development. Both effects may confer significant psychological benefit.
2 ACTH deficiency: Hydrocortisone is required in dosages carefully tailored to match the needs of the individual.
3 TSH deficiency: Thyroxine is indicated.

THYROID DISEASE

Thyrotoxicosis

Thyrotoxics may be treated by drugs, surgery and radioiodine therapy. Surgery has the best results in terms of permanent cure; oral radioiodine therapy is simple but commonly followed by hypothyroidism, though often only after many years (60 % at 10 years). A prolonged period of drug therapy (i.e. 18 months) has a 50 % permanent remission rate, the remainder relapsing. Current practice is varied. In general, surgery is avoided in children and radioiodine restricted to the eldery. In the young and middle-aged adult, a prolonged course of drug is often used, to be followed up by surgery should relapse ensue.

Propranolol (p.93)
Many of the distressing symptoms of thyrotoxicosis are due to increased sympathetic activity which can be successfully blocked with propranolol. It does not modify the activity of the gland and is in no way curative.

Thiourea derivitives (e.g. carbimazole)
Pharmacological action: Thioureas block the incorporation of iodine into the precursors of thyroxine. Thyroxine and tri-iodothyronine secretion is reduced.
    Toxicity: (a) Hypersensitivity. Rashes are common. Aplastic anaemia and agranulocytosis are rare but serious. (b) Goitre. Continued extra-thyroidal stimulation of the gland predisposes to goitre in the presence of thioureas.

Perchlorate
Pharmacological action: Reduces the ability of the gland to concentrate iodide by interfering with the "iodide trap".
    Toxicity: Rashes are rare but the risk of aplastic anaemia is greater than with thiourea drugs.

Potassium iodide
Pharmacological action. Although the oldest remedy in hyperthyroidism, its action remains unknown. Observed effects are symptomatic improvement, and reduction in vascularity of the gland (the latter often welcomed by the thyroid surgeon).

Hypothyroidism Whether due to pituitary disease or primary thyroid failure, the treatment of hypothyroidism is by replacement therapy with thyroxine.

PARATHYROID DISEASE

The main function of parathyroid hormone is to regulate the concentration of calcium in the body fluids. In health, its secretion is regulated by the serum calcium level (direct negative feed-back).

Hyperparathyroidism

The definitive treatment is resection of parathyroid tissue, although intravenous infusion of phosphate is sometimes used in a hypercalcaemic crisis.

Hypoparathyroidism

Parathyroid insufficiency is characterized by tetany and psychological changes due to low serum calcium levels. Replacement therapy with parathyroid extract is both expensive and unreliable. Instead, Vitamin D is used.

Vitamin D (see also p.192)

The collective name for a group of similar compounds.

Pharmacological action
Vitamin D has three principal actions on:
1   the intestinal absorption of calcium;
2   the calcification of bone;
3   the renal excretion of calcium.

In the absence of parathyroid hormone (hypoparathyroidism), Vitamin D therapy can maintain normal serum calcium levels and normal bone structure provided that dietary calcium is adequate.

Kinetics
Adequately (50 %) absorbed orally; this is a fat-soluble vitamin and normal bile production is essential to its absorption. It is metabolized by several tissues (the metabolites are probably responsible for its pharmacological activity).

Unwanted effects
In correct dosage, Vitamin D is non-toxic. The effects of overdosage are discussed elsewhere.

ADRENAL DISEASE

Adrenal Hyperfunction

Adrenal hyperfunction is treated surgically, whether due to pituitary or adrenal adenoma.

Adrenal Insufficiency

The adrenal cortex secretes glucocorticoids, mineralocorticoids, and small quantities of sex steroids (p.156). Mineralocorticoids (aldosterone) are independent of pituitary stimulus. Intrinsic adrenal failure (Addison's disease) requires replacement therapy with both a glucocorticoid and mineralocorticoid; in adrenal failure caused by pituitary disease, only the glucocorticoid is usually necessary.

Replacement Therapy

Glucocorticoid
Cortisone or hydrocortisone are suitable.
(Cortisone is converted by the body to hydrocortisone).
    Physiological action: (see p.157).
    Kinetics: Discussed in detail on p.156. Correct replacement dosages do not produce the serious side-effects characteristic of therapeutic doses (p.159).

Mineralocorticoid:
Fludrocortisone (synthetic) is used.
    Physiological action: Regulation of sodium balance and extra-cellular fluid volume.
    Kinetics: Fludrocortisone is the only orally effective mineralocorticoid.
    Unwanted effects: Nil in correct replacement dosage.
Excess may produce Sodium retention with oedema. Insufficient

quantities result in hypovolaemia, haemoconcentration and fall in blood pressure.

Notes
In the event of major stress — infections, surgery, anaesthesia, trauma, heart attack, serious emotional disturbances — the dose of hydrocortisone should be doubled. In the most acute situations, hydrocortisone should be injected for immediate effect (see under Adrenal Crisis p.160).

All steroid-dependent patients should be encouraged to carry a steroid card stating steroid dosage and general practitioner's name. Ideally they should wear an engraved bracelet.

OVARIAN DISEASE

Ovarian dysfunction may be primary or result from pituitary disease. Amenorrhoea is not necessarily a sign of pituitary or ovarian disease: chronic debilitating illness, metobolic upset, physchological disturbance and other endocrine diseases are common causes and probably interfere functionally with the hypothalamic-pituitary-ovarian axis.

In the case of ovarian failure, secondary sexual characteristics (but not fertility) may be maintained or restored with cyclical use of oestrogens and progestogens. These are discussed under the next heading, Oral Contraceptives.

ORAL CONTRACEPTIVES

About two million women in Britain are now 'on the pill' regularly, indicating its wide acceptability and also its importance as a drug. Pregnancy, although physiological, carries a high incidence of morbidity and rarely mortality. All other methods of contraception are less effective, and since lack of effectiveness is measured in pregnancies, the pill is also the safest method.

Pharmacological Control of Conception

1   Combination of oestrogen and progestogen throughout cycle.
2   Sequential use of oestrogen in the first half and a combination of oestrogen and progestogen in the latter half of the cycle.
3   Progestogen alone through cycle.

Oestrogen:

Oestrogen is a generic term for a group of similar substances. Oestrone and oestradiol are naturally occurring; vast numbers of synthetic preparations exist.

Pharmacological action
1   Suppression of release of pituitary gonadotrophins; the ovarian follicle fails to ripen and ovulation is prevented.
2   Continued maintenance of a proliferative endometrium.
Menstruation is suppressed or delayed.
3   Maintance of a healthy vaginal epithelium.
4   Mild mineralocorticoid action.

Kinetics
Oral absorption is complete. Natural oestrogens are rapidly inactivated: synthetic preparations are only slowly metabolized and are therefore therapeutically effective when taken orally.

Unwanted effects
· Exacerbation of chronic marginal gingivitis (cf pregnancy gingivitis).
· Nausea (cf morning sickness in early pregnancy).
· Breakthrough bleeding. Despite continued use of oestrogen throughout the cycle, troublesome and unpredictable shedding of the endometrium may occur.
· Fluid retention; may be sufficient to cause oedema and even precipitate heart failure in those predisposed.
· Impairment of carbohydrate tolerance; latent diabetes may appear and overt diabetes is commonly aggravated.
· Hypertension (p.72). Aggravation of existing hypertension is common.
· Amenorrhoea following withdrawal of oestrogens (due to the prolonged suppression of pituitary gonadotrophins).
· Thrombosis; current evidence suggests a significantly increased incidence of venous thrombosis and pulmonary embolism amongst those taking oestrogen-containing contraceptives.

Progestogen

Pharmacological action
· Cervical mucus glands: the normally abundant watery secretion of the cervix becomes thick, scanty and non-conducive to the passage of sperms. This is the main contraceptive action of progestogens.
· Endometrium; artificial prolongation of the secretory phase (latter half

of cycle) by continuous administration of progestogens results in atrophy of the endometrial cells; normal appearances can be restored by adding oestrogen.

Kinetics
Oral absorption is prompt and inactivation by the liver rapid.

Unwanted effects
Outwith pregnancy, side-effects are very rare in contrast with the adverse reactions attributable to oestrogen preparations.

PANCREATIC ISLET CELLS

The islets of Langerhans in the pancreas possess two types of cell; the α-cell secretes glucagon and the β-cell insulin.

Glucagon

In therapeutic doses glucagon will raise a reduced blood sugar. Physiologically it has several complex actions which are only now coming to light. It will not be further considered here.

Insulin

Action of Insulin
In health, insulin secretion varies according to the blood sugar level, rising after a carbohydrate meal and falling once the carbohydrate absorption has ceased. This phenomenon can be observed indirectly by giving a fasting patient 50 g of oral glucose and measuring serially the blood sugar levels.
    This glucose tolerance test normally produces a shallow curve, with a return to the fasting blood sugar level within two hours. Insulin acts primarily by facilitating the peripheral uptake of blood glucose into muscle, fat and liver cells. Its secondary actions are best described in terms of the disturbance which results from insulin deficiency. These are:
· Elevated blood sugar. The glucose tolerance curve of insulin deficiency has an abnormally high peak and the return to fasting levels may take several hours, suggesting that the rate of blood sugar clearance is diminished. Thirst and polyuria result from osmotic action of high blood sugar concentrations on the kidney.
· Ketosis. Glucose-deprived cells revert to fat as a source of energy. One of the end-products of fat catabolism is a group of keto-acids which are toxic when present in excess.

· Protein breakdown. Protein is broken down to replenish glycogen stores in the liver and muscle. Wasting occurs.

ISLET CELL DISEASE

Functioning β-cell adenomas (insulinomas) rarely occur and cause hypoglycaemia through insulin excess. Treatment is ideally surgical.

Insulin deficiency is far more common. The deficiency may be absolute; alternatively insulin antagonists may be present in the blood which reduce insulin *activity* rather than the plasma level of insulin.

Diabetes Mellitus (Mel, mellis (L); honey)

Diabetes is defined in terms of abnormalities in the glucose tolerance curve noted above. When blood sugar exceeds 7.5-10 mmol/l the kidney can no longer absorb all its filtered glucose and glycosuria results, often the first sign of diabetes. Three principal diabetic syndromes exist:

1 Acute (juvenile) onset. Generally presents within the first 50 years of life and is characterized by an absolute lack of insulin. The onset is usually sudden and owing to complete lack of insulin activity, ketosis is a prominent complication.

2 Sub-acute (maturity) onset. Maturity onset diabetes usually develops in the second half of life. Because some insulin activity is usually present, ketosis is seldom a problem; the onset is gradual and management usually simpler. Insulin is required only in a minority.

3 Secondary diabetes. Growth hormone, glucocorticoid steroids and adrenaline antagonize the action of insulin. Elevated blood sugar levels, abnormal tolerance curves and glycosuria are thus commonly found in acromegaly, Cushing's disease, phaeodromocytoma and thyrotoxicosis. In addition, simple obesity causes insulin antagonism, a fact of major relevance to the management of many cases of maturity onset diabetes.

Principles of Clinical Management

Healthy people secrete insulin in direct response to carbohydrate intake. Many diabetics depend on a regular dose of insulin and this must match or be matched by a regular intake of carbohydrate.

Diet

First, the diabetician (usually in conjunction with a dietician), will judge the calorie needs of his patient. Obviously a petite sedentary secretary has calorie requirements very different from those of a muscular labourer. Calories are available in the diet as fat, protein and carbohydrate. Only carbohydrate requires insulin. To be palatable a 2000 calorie diet should contain about 200 g carbohydrate (a 1500 calorie diet, 150 g, and so on). Provided his insulin dose is appropriate to the 200 g of carbohydrate, the patient can arrange the fat and protein content to his liking. If he eats too much fat or protein, he would simply gain weight without acute disturbance of his diabetic control (in the long term, however, weight gain would increase his insulin needs).

Insulin

Having established an acceptable eating pattern with his patient, (and acceptability is the single most important factor), the physician can begin to tailor an insulin regime accordingly. The success of the regime is assessed by regular blood sugar estimations; once stabilized, the patient can monitor his own urine sugar, using a home-testing kit.

Insulins are available in rapidly-acting soluble form or in suspensions with various durations of action. Two points are important:

1   Insulin regimes are never perfect; the optimum regime merely represents the best compromise.

2   Some textbooks tabulate the times of onset and duration of action of various insulins, as if tight limits existed. Experience suggests immense variations in response, particularly to long-acting insulins.

Pharmacological action

In diabetes, insulin reverses the hyperglycaemia and ketosis noted above, in addition to restoring to normal the metabolism of fat and protein.

Kinetics

Insulin is destroyed by gastric enzymes and must be administered parenterally. It is degraded by the liver. Its onset, peak and offset of action depend upon the site of injection (s.c., i.m., or i.v.) and upon the preparation used.

Toxicity

1   Hypersensitivty. Rashes are uncommon. Insulin is a foreign protein, and sometimes the emergence of insulin antibodies renders a particular preparation ineffective. The use of an alternative source of insulin may restore effective control.

2   Fat atrophy (lipodystrophy) is a local complication of repeated injections at the same site.

Oral hypoglycaemic agents

Oral antidiabetic drugs are only effective in patients who lack the tendency to become ketotic; this implies the presence of some endogenous insulin activity and includes the majority of maturity onset diabetics. Two groups of oral hypoglycaemic drugs are in common usage:

Sulphonylureas
A group of sulphonamide-derived drugs.
   Pharmacological action: Stimulation of insulin release from pancreatic β-cells (therefore ineffective in situations of total insulin deficiency).

Biguanide drugs
Pharmacological action: This is uncertain but biguanides appear to act principally by augmenting the action of insulin on cell membranes (this also applies to injected insulin). They also supress appetite.

Preparation of the Diabetic for General Anaesthesia

The aid of the physician must be sought in preparing an insulin-dependent diabetic for general anaesthesia.

The insulin-dependent diabetic

It is essential to establish the degree of insulin dependence (i.e. tendency or otherwise to ketosis — insulin dosage is not a good indication).

(a) Major Elective procedures (requiring in-patient care)
Unstable diabetics. Admit to hospital 2-3 days before operation. A suitable regime is to stabilize the patient on soluble insulin bd. Both insulin and food should be omitted on the day of operation and the procedure carried out first thing in the morning. A blood sugar should be checked prior to anaesthetic and 2-3 hr after operation whereupon adjustments in subsequent insulin dosage can be made. If the patient is unable to take solid food, the hospital dietician should be requested to supply the appropriate carbohydrate in soft or liquid form.
   Severe diabetics (strong tendency to ketosis). Prepare as above but 1 hr prior to operation give 40 % the patient's normal morning dose of insulin in soluble form and inject 25 g of dextrose (as a 10 % solution) i.v. A constant i.v. infusion of dextrose will normally be required if the operation

is prolonged beyond 1 hr. Post-operative measurement of blood sugar will guide subsequent management.

(b) Emergency procedures (i.e. facial trauma requiring immediate attention)
Small subcutaneous doses (10-20 IU) of soluble insulin should be given 3-4 hourly or occasionally more frequently to maintain blood sugar below 15 mmol/l.

(c) Minor procedures (out-patient care)
The case should be first on the morning list. Breakfast and insulin can be delayed until after treatment.

The mild diabetic (diet alone or diet + oral hypoglycaemic drug)

Omit both food and drug on the morning of operation and administer the drug after recovery from anaesthetic.

Conclusion

The risk to avoid at all costs is hypoglycaemia during general anaesthesia.

Local anaesthesia
Stress may raise the blood sugar of insulin-dependent diabetics but the effect should only be transient and very unlikely to present a problem.

Insulin Reaction

Excessive insulin (or more commonly insufficient food) may lead to hypo-glycaemic coma in the diabetic. The manifestations are those of high adrenergic activity (*cf.* thyrotoxicosis) followed by failing consciousness. The patient becomes sweaty, tremulous and begins to lose concentration. The skin is clammy and the pulse thin and rapid. Oral or intravenous (up to 50 %) glucose should be given as appropriate.

4.13 PAIN

Simple analgesics
Salicylates
   Aspirin (acetyl salicylic acid)

Soluble aspirin
Enteric coated aspirin
Aniline derivatives
Paracetamol
Phenacetin

Opiate analgesics
Restricted
Morphine
Diamorphine
Pethidine
Papavaretum
Methadone
Non-restricted
Dihydrocodeine
Pentazocine
Codeine

Opiate antagonists
Nalorphine
Naloxone

MECHANISMS IN THE APPRECIATION OF PAIN

Pain is one of the commonest associations of disease yet one of the most difficult to assess. Two factors operate: intensity of the causal stimulus and the emotional reaction to it. These factors act independently and variably so that the best approach to relief is not always through analgesia alone (suggestion is frequently successful).

Stimulus

Pain is a protective reflex and in health usually implies tissue damage. Pain stimuli are probably mediated through chemical transmitters, produced at the site of the pain, and which trigger nerve impulses.

The Receptor

The original concept of receptors individually subserving different modalities of sensation has long been challenged. Melzack & Wall (1965) postulated the currently accepted Gate Control Theory.

Different sensory modalities, among them pain, produce different patterns of receptor response — in terms of threshold, peak sensitivity, adaptation rate etc. The many permutations of these variables permit a wide variety of impulse patterns to be produced.

Peripheral nerves and Spinal Cord

Peripheral sensory nerves may be of small or large diameter and both can stimulate central transmission (T) Cells in the spinal cord which activate cerebral systems responsible for perception of the original stimulus. This arrangement is however modulated by a gate which if closed will prevent activation of T Cells by peripheral impulses. The gate is positioned by two influences — (1) the relative impulse load between large and small diameter peripheral nerves, and (2) central(cerebral) control. The effects of large and small fibre stimulation tend to oppose one another; if stimulation is prolonged, large fibres adapt and permit an increase in T Cell output by opening the gate. An increase in large fibre activity produced by vibration or scratching for instance, reduces adaptation and the gate closes.

Central Control Trigger

Conduction through the gate is also influenced by facilitation from higher cerebral control. Rapidly conveyed information about the external stimulus is passed to the brain, processed, and the appropriate impulses returned to the spinal cord in order to position the gate accordingly. It is likely that factors such as past experience, emotional status and environmental situation will influence this facilitation pathway and permit or prevent the passage of pain impulse.

Action System

Pain, its interpretation and its associated responses are the result of complex interactions triggered when the T Cell output exceeds a critical level. Location of source, magnitude and character of the impulses are assessed and in the light of past experience, evasive action taken as appropriate. The reaction to suden, severe and unexpected pain involves basic defensive reflexes common to all beings. The cortical reaction to chronic pain varies from fortitude to despair and it is this aspect of the medical approach to pain which provides the greatest therapeutic challenge.

THE ROLE OF DRUGS IN THE CONTROL OF PAIN

Many simple analgesics act peripherally in reducing the frequency or modifying the pattern of pain impulses. Anti-inflammatory drugs (p.150) are usually either weak (e.g. salicylate) or lacking (corticosteroids) in intrinsic analgesic activity, but act rather by suppressing the inflammatory stimulus to pain.

Strong analgesics usually possess a major central component to their action which greatly alters the cerebral response to pain as well as reducing its intensity by adjustment of the gate. Such drugs are usually reserved for severe visceral pain and their use is limited by important side effects.

The contribution of an understanding, reassuring and sympathetic dental attendant cannot be evaluated in physiological terms but it is as important in the control of pain as any individual drug. In some cases, reassurance can reduce pain intensity to acceptable levels without recourse to drugs.

SIMPLE (NON-NARCOTIC) ANALGESICS

SALICYLATES

The active salicylate ion is mildly analgesic and has a principally peripheral action. It has no influence on the psychic reaction to pain and is most effective in mild pain of somatic (i.e. non-visceral) origin. At higher doses salicylates also have strong anti-inflammatory and antipyretic actions. Kinetics and toxicity are discussed elswhere (p.152).

Presentation
Aspirin (acetylsalicylic acid) 300 mg tablet
Soluble aspirin (ASA/citric acid/calcium carbonate) 300 mg tablet
Enteric coated aspirin - aspirin 300 mg sugar-coated tablet

Administration
Although Salicylate is the most commonly used mild analgesic, it is more specifically indicated in painful inflammatory conditions (see p.152) such as rheumatoid arthritis; the dose for mild analgesia is 300-600 mg q.i.d, that for inflammation between 3 and 4 g daily. If pure analgesia only is sought, Paracetamol is a safer drug.

ANILINE DERIVATIVES

Because of their derivation the members of this group are sometimes called the coal-tar analgesics. They include paracetamol (acetaminophen).

Paracetamol and Phenacetin

Analgesia
A peripheral action is postulated. The effect is restricted to moderate pain such as headache, toothache and integumental (non-arthritic) pains, and lasts 3-4 hours following a single dose.

Antipyresis
Aniline derivatives have *no* anti-inflammatory action.

Kinetics
Both are rapidly and completely absorbed from the G.I. Tract and are not strongly plasma protein-bound. Both drugs are completely metabolized by liver enzymes; the major metabolite of phenacetin is paracetamol but phenacetin is pharmacologically active in its own right. Barbiturates may reduce the plasma levels of aniline drugs by enzyme-induction (p.171).

Toxicity
1   Most important neither preparation is a gastric irritant (*cf* Salicylate).
2   Habituation. Habituation to these drugs is probably a far more serious problem than is commonly realized. Withdrawal symptoms are mild — restlessness and excitement are the most common. The most important result of habituation is renal damage: analgesic nephropathy.
3   Analgesic nephropathy. Regular daily consumption of phenacetin (and probably also paracetamol) over a period of years may produce severe irreversible and often fatal interstitial nephritis. The degree of damage is related to the cumulative consumption which may amount to many kilograms.
4   Methaemoglobinaemia and haemolytic anaemia may occur, particularly in acute overdosage.
5   Acute overdosage. Overdosage with 10 g or more (20 tablets) of paracetamol is likely to cause acute hepatic necrosis. Many cases are fatal.

Paracetamol

Presentation
Tablets 500 mg.

Administration
500 mg-1 g q.i.d. for mild somatic pain. In the absence of inflammatory disease, paracetamol is as effective and certainly safer than aspirin.

Phenacetin

Presentation
As a constituent of many proprietary pain-killers, commonly in combination with aspirin and codeine.

Administration
There is no evidence that either phenacetin or its combinants are any more effective when formulated together. The simplest advice is to avoid fixed drug combinations.

Note

Indole and pyrazolone derivatives (indomethacin, phenylbutazone) are considered primarily anti-inflammatory drugs and are discussed on pages 154-5.

OPIATE (NARCOTIC) ANALGESICS AND RELATED DRUGS

Opium is a crude mixture of related alkaloids derived from the dried poppy seed (*Papaver somniferum*) and has been known to medicine at least since Egyptian times. Morphine and codeine are the two important alkaloids in use today. Noscapine and papaverine are occasionally used in purified forms as anaesthetic pre-medicants. Tincture of Opium has long since disappeared. With the purification of individual alkaloids have appeared a number of synthetic narcotics. The word narcosis simply means sleep.

Morphine (representative of the opiates)

Pharmacological actions
CNS
    (a) Depressant: analgesia, respiratory depression, sleep (narcosis).
    (b) Stimulant: meiosis (constant sign — pin-point pupils), vomiting (cerebral action), convulsions.
    (c) Mood change: most commonly euphoria and sense of detachment but occasionally anxiety and agitation.
    (d) Addiction.
Smooth muscle stimulant
    Spasm (colic).
    Analgesia is the outstanding therapeutic action of morphine and may be

attributed to a number of independent mechanisms:
· Elevation of pain threshold.
· Modified psychic reaction to perceived pain.
· Sleep induction — narcosis.
   Morphine has no peripheral effects on pain reception. Respiratory
depression is dose-related. The respiratory centre becomes less responsive
to the plasma pCo_2 and the cough reflex is depressed. Therapeutic doses
of morphine have little effect on the CVS. The problems of addiction and
morphine withdrawal are discussed on pages 212-3.

Tolerance
A feature of all opiate analgesics. When morphine is used over many weeks
the dose required to produce a constant effect may increase 20-fold. The
same is true for the addict as for the patient receiving morphine for
legitimate reasons.

Overdose
Death in overdosage results from respiratory depression: Anoxia causes
circulatory failure. It is essential to identify (firstly) the drug as morphine
(since a specific antagonist is available) and (secondly) acute overdosage in
an addict. In the latter, complete withdrawal of the drug may precipitate a
withdrawal syndrome.

Kinetics
Opiates are readily absorbed from the G.I. tract although greater effect is
usually obtained with parenteral administration.

Toxicity
Respiratory depression can be significant in therapeutic dosage:
(a) where obstructive airways disease is present;
(b) in drug interaction.
   Many drugs exaggerate the cerebral depressant effects of morphia
(phenothiazines, MAO inhibitors, tricyclic antidepressant drugs).
   CNS Effects: vomiting, dizziness and dysphoria. These are common and
indicate the desirability of giving an anti-emetic with the morphine. Convulsions are rare.

Diamorphine (heroin)

Diamorphine (diacetylmorphine) is a semisynthetic opiate; it is rapidly
hydrolysed to morphine following administration, and many contend that
morphine is the pharmacologically active agent in heroin. Its actions are
similar to those of morphine although some claim (controversially) that it

is less liable to induce nausea, produces greater euphoria, and is more strongly addictive. Diamorphine is the more potent.

Pethidine

Pethidine was developed first as a spasmolytic drug on account of its atropinic action. It is structurally dissimilar from the opiates but has selective actions in common with morphine:

1   Analgesia; its potency lies between that of codeine and morphine.
2   Respiratory depression (the cause of death in overdose).
3   Vomiting.
4   Dependence and tolerance (psychic effects of detachment and euphoria are less marked).
5   Competitive antagonism by nalorphine and naloxone.
     It differs importantly in the following respects:
1   It is effective orally.
2   Is ineffective as cough-suppressant and influences gut motility far less.
3   Does not stimulate the oculomotor nucleus — meiosis is not a sign of pethidine administration.
4   Lesser hypnotic effects.

Specific toxic effects
1   Interaction with other drugs: Delirium or convulsions may occur when given concurrently with MAO inhibitors. Respiratory depression may become a serious problem in patient already taking phenothiazines.
2   Hypotension: pethidine has a more potent hypotensive action than morphine.

Methadone

Pharmacological actions similar to those of morphine. The principal differences are:
· effective orally;
· significantly less hypnotic.
Methadone shares the same problems with morphine — respiratory depression, vomiting following administration and addiction. Addiction however is milder with slower onset and less distressing withdrawal effects.

Dihydrocodeine

Pharmacological actions
1   Analgesia with sedation: the degree of analgesia is similar to that obtained from morphine but it is non-narcotic.

2   Lacks significant cough-suppressant action, is non-addictive, and does not cause respiratory depression in therapeutic doses.

Toxicity
1   Nausea and giddiness — probably dose related.
2   Asthmatic attacks: asthma may be worsened in those predisposed and the drug should be avoided.
3   Constipation.

Presentation
Injection 50 mg in 1 ml
Tablets 30 mg
Elixir 10 mg in 5 ml.

Administration
Dihydrocodeine offers moderate analgesia (between that of codeine and morphine) without significant sedative or hypnotic effect. It is fully effective when given orally but is not recommended for children. It can be considered non-addictive. The dose is 30-60 mg according to need.

Pentazocine

Introduced as a non-addictive analgesic to replace morphine. In practice it has similar analgesic efficacy to morphine but lacks the influence on psychic reaction to pain which singles out morphine as a unique drug.
    Pentazocine is a synthetic opiate antagonist which like nalorphine (qv) can precipitate withdrawal symptoms in the morphine addict. It has only very weak addictive properties of its own.
    Pentazocine is well absorbed orally and is effective for 3-4 hr following administration. It is metabolized in the liver.

Side-effects
Sedation, giddiness and nausea are the commonest; recent reports suggest that hallucinatory effects may also be common, particularly in the elderly. Overdosage effects (mainly depression of the CNS) may be reversed by *naloxone* and not by nalorphine.

Presentation
Injection Ampoules 30 mg/ml in 1 ml or 2 ml.
Capsules 50 mg
Tablets 15 mg
Suppositories 50 mg.

Administration

In moderate to severe pain, pentazocine offers analgesia without fear of addiction. It should be avoided in those with chronic obstructive airways disease and must not be used in patients receiving opiates on a regular basis. Adequate analgesia can usually be obtained with 30-60 mg 4-hourly. The suppository provides nocturnal relief of pain.

Codeine

Less potent than morphine as an analgesic (about 20 % as effective) and far less liable to produce side effects. Most important it is non-narcotic (large doses may produce excitability) and non-addictive.

Clinical toxicity is rare and codeine is not liable to abuse.

Presentation
Tablets 15 mg, *30 mg*, 60 mg
Linctus 15 mg in 5 ml
Paediatric linctus 3 mg in 5 ml.

Administration
Large doses produce analgesia similar to that of morphine but in therapeutic dosage it is a little more potent than aspirin. Unlike morphine it is fully effective when given orally.

In addition to analgesia codeine is useful as a cough-suppressant and anti-diarrhoeal agent. (Unwanted constipation may accompany its use as a cough-suppressant linctus). Codeine compound (Codeine Co.) contains more paracetamol than codeine and should not be used as a constipant or cough suppressant.

OPIATE ANTAGONISTS

Antagonists are used to reverse the acute effects of opiates. Traditionally nalorphine or levallorphan has been used but more recently naloxone has been shown to have several important advantages.

Nalorphine

Two important actions:
1   Reversal of respiratory depression following acute opiate overdosage.
2   Precipitation of withdrawal symptoms if used injudiciously in the addict. Whilst this action is undesirable in the treatment of acute

overdosage in the addict, it can serve the useful diagnostic purpose of "unmasking" physical dependence on morphine or heroin where addiction is suspected.

Nalorphine is only effective in antagonizing the action of pure opiates (e.g. morphine, heroin, methadone) and may in excessive dosage itself lead to respiratory depression.

Naloxone

Action: a specific opiate antagonist which differs advantageously from Nalorphine in several respects:
1   No intrinsic respiratory depressant action (nor sedative, meiotic or psychomimetic effects).
2   Effective in reversing the action of pentazocine as well as the pure opiate drugs.
3   Between 10 and 20 times more potent than Nalorphine in counteracting narcotic-induced respiratory depression.
4   The chronic administration of Naloxone does not lead to tolerance of its effect, as is the case with Nalorphine.

4.14   INFLAMMATION

Simple anti-inflammatory drugs:
Salicylates
    Aspirin
    Soluble aspirin
    Enteric-coated aspirin
Naproxen

Pyrazolone derivatives
    Phenylbutazone
    Oxyphenbutazone
Indole derivatives
    Indomethacin
Anthranilic acid derivatives
    Mefenamic acid
    Flufenamic acid
Sodium aurothiomalate (gold)

Adrenal corticosteroids
    Hydrocortisone
    Prednisolone
    Betamethasone and dexamethasone
    ACTH

Antihistamines
  Promethazine
  Chlorpheniramine
Note
Pain may be a primary symptom (i.e. traumatic pain) or it may be secondary to inflammation. Inflammatory pain will respond to specific anti-inflammatory drugs, primary pain requires only analgesics. The distinction is important because although some of the drugs cited have both analgesic and anti-inflammatory properties, anti-inflammatory drugs as a group are undoubtedly more toxic than the simple (non-narcotic) analgesics.

THE INFLAMMATORY RESPONSE

The inflammatory reaction is an essential vital process; in some cases the maintenance of life may depend upon it. Like other vital processes, however, inflammation may become aberrant and may prove more harmful to the body than the stimulus which produced it.

Wright (1958) has defined inflammation as a process by which cells and exudate accumulate in irritated tissues and *usually* tend to protect them from further damage. Such is the case with infections which are localized by inflammation and which subsequently either resolve spontaneously or by rupture (e.g. abscess). Harmful inflammation may arise in a wide variety of conditions (such as those known collectively as the collagen or connective tissue diseases). Examples in dentistry are the dermatoses which may involve the oral mucosa, such as lichen planus and Beçet's syndrome.

Even the protective inflammatory responses may become harmful in certain situations: while inflamed skin can swell freely without exerting local pressures, an inflamed dental pulp has no room for expansion and the resulting pressure (apart from producing excruciating pain) may so jeopardise the local blood supply as to result in pulp necrosis.

Physiologically, inflammation is a complex reaction triggered by tissue damage which may result from traumatic, chemical or immunological insult. Early on, inflammation (from whatever cause) is characterized by oedema, fibrin deposition, phagocytic activity and capillary dilatation. This stage frequently gives rise to considerable pain. Both the pain and inflammatory reaction are thought to be mediated by the local synthesis of complex chemicals known as prostaglandins. Later manifestations of inflammation include fibroblastic proliferation and collagen deposition.

THE ROLE OF ANTI-INFLAMMATORY DRUGS

Anti-inflammatory drugs are used primarily to alleviate the pain resulting from destructive inflammatory reactions. They may also be helpful in controlling the symptoms of an aggressive though protective inflammatory response. There are three broad drug groups:

1   The simple anti-inflammatory analgesics such as aspirin, phenylbutazone, indomethacin etc, which act peripherally, probably by antagonising the synthesis of prostaglandins.

2   Corticosteroids such as prednisolone, which prevent both the early and late expressions of the inflammatory reaction. Steroids are thought to stabilize the cellular lysosomal sacs which are otherwise broken down by the inflammatory stimulus to release the enzymes and other mediators responsible for the manifestations of inflammation. It must be emphasised that steroids are non-selective and will equally suppress protective responses should the patient develop concurrent infection. Neither do they influence the underlying cause of the inflammation; clinically their effect is potent but palliative.

3   Antihistamines — histamine release is a feature of the anaphylactic reaction (p.194) and amongst other substances it is responsible for the characteristic wheal and flare reaction of urticaria and its more serious manifestation, angioneurotic oedema. Antihistamine drugs can suppress these particular responses and may therefore be considered anti-inflammatory.

Note
It is desirable in most circumstances not to eliminate, but rather to modify the excessive or aberrant inflammatory reaction and appropriate drugs are widely used in medicine today.

INDIVIDUAL DRUGS

SIMPLE ANTI-INFLAMMATORY AGENTS

Salicylates

Derived originally from the willow bark (Salix alba). A number of synthetic preparations are now available but all depend for their activity on the release of salicylic acid within the body. Aspirin is but one of many synthetic salicylates which differ mainly in potency; even the significance of this is doubtful in practice.

Pharmacological actions
Anti-inflammatory. Specific in suppressing the polyarthritis of acute rheumatic fever; similarly effective in rheumatoid arthritis and in minor

connective-tissue inflammations associated with acute viral diseases.
Analgesia (p.143). Alleviate certain types of mild pain.
Antipyresis. Reduce elevated body temperature by a central action on the
temperature-regulating centre of the hypothalamus.
Uricosuric effects. In large doses (3 g+per day) Salicylates encourage the
renal excretion of uric acid though in low doses (less than 1.5 g/day), the
effect is reversed.

Kinetics

Well absorbed from the stomach where the high pH gradient between
gastric juice and the interior of mucosal cells encourages the rapid absorption of an acidic drug. (Enteric-coated preparations of aspirin are absorbed
in the small intestine where the high intracellular concentration of the
drug, which accounts for damage to gastric mucosa, does not occur).

Presentation

Aspirin (acetylsalicylic acid) 300 mg tablet
Soluble aspirin (ASA/citric acid/calcium carbonate) 300 mg tablet.
Enteric-coated aspirin — Aspirin 300 mg sugar-coated tablet.

Aspirin is the drug of choice in the treatment of rheumatoid arthritis
and related syndromes. It is effective in relieving pain from minor dental
and periodontal inflammations, when a smaller dose is sufficient.

Gastric irritation limits the acceptability of high-dose aspirin regimens
in a large number of cases. Soluble aspirin may be better tolerated but is
less potent; Enteric coated aspirin is designed to break up beyond the
stomach. Some patients are unable to tolerate aspirin whatever its formulation.

Side-effects and contra-indications

1 Nausea and dyspepsia — heartburn is common.
2 G.I. haemorrhage — a common cause of admission to hospital yet it
must be considered a rare association in terms of the vast national
consumption of aspirin. Chronic G.I. blood loss of a few ml/day is far
commoner and usually asymptomatic.
3 Hypersensitivity — Aspirin is one of the commonest causes of drug-
induced urticaria. Asthma is less common and anaphylactic shock rare.
Aspirin is contra-indicated in those with a past history of upper G.I.,
bleeding, dyspepsia, gastric surgery, bleeding diathesis and in those taking
anticoagulants.

Naproxen

A non-steroidal anti-inflammatory agent unrelated to any other compounds currently in use. Like aspirin it has strong anti-inflammatory

properties and is both analgesic and antipyretic.

Kinetics
Well-absorbed orally. It is strongly protein-bound and may displace drugs such as phenytoin, warfarin and sulphonamides, increasing their free plasma concentrations to toxic levels.

Toxicity
Gastro-intestinal bleeding — reports are rare but the drug should preferably be withheld where bleeding is a potential problem.

Allergic reactions, mainly skin urticaria and angio-oedema. Naproxen should be avoided in atopic "allergic" individuals.

Pyrazolone derivatives

Phenylbutazone

Pharmacological actions
Powerful anti-inflammatory agent
Uricosuric in high dose
Weak analgesic.

Kinetics
Well absorbed from the gut. Phenylbutazone gives rise to two important types of drug interaction:
1   Competitive protein binding: Phenylbutazone is 98 % protein bound; it will displace many other drugs from plasma proteins, resulting in exaggerated responses to apparently normal dosage. Such is the case with Warfarin (over-anticoagulation and potentially serious bleeding) and sulphonylureas (excess hypoglycaemic action and possiblity of coma).
2   Enzyme induction: the induction of hepatic drug metabolizing enzymes by phenylbutazone may reduce the expected response to some other drugs given concurrently: by the same token phenylbutazone induces its own metabolism and doses in excess of 500 mg daily do not significantly increase the plasma level but may increase toxicity attributable to metabolites.

Toxicity
1   Blood dyscrasias — phenylbutazone is probably the commonest cause of drug-induced aplastic anaemia. Agranulocytosis may occur alone.
2   Gastro-intestinal upset and haemorrhage similar to that induced by aspirin.
3   Oedema — interference with the mechanism for the renal excretion of sodium may result in oedema.

Oxyphenbutazone

Marketed as a drug in its own right although it is the active product of phenylbutazone metabolism. Its kinetics and toxicity are similar to those of phenylbutazone.

Indole derivatives

Indomethacin

Pharmacological actions
Anti-inflammatory — potent.
Antipyresis — more potent than that of aspirin.
Analgesia — weak.

Kinetics
Complete gastro-intestinal absorption.

Toxicity
1   Gastro-intestinal: anorexia, nausea, mucosal ulceration, haemorrhage and abdominal pain.
2   CNS: Severe frontal headache, vertigo and confusion; occasionally depression and hallucination.
3   Marrow — neutropenia and rarely aplastic anaemia.
4   Hypersensitivity — rashes, itching, urticaria, allergic asthma.

Presentation
Capsules 25 mg, 50 mg.
Oral suspension 25 mg in 5 ml.

Administration
Indicated in inflammations which have failed to respond to salicylates. It has proved effective in oral inflammations caused by systemic collagen diseases.
    Indomethacin should not be given to children.

Anthranilic acid derivatives

Mefenamic acid and Flufenamic acid

Anti-inflammatory, antipyretic and mildly analgesic; potency similar to aspirin.

Toxicity
Gastro-intestinal irritation, diarrhoea and maculo-papular rashes are the commonest. Mefenamic acid may displace warfarin from protein-binding sites and increase the plasma prothrombin time accordingly.

Gold (Sodium aurothiomalate)

Pharmacological action
Anti-inflammatory. The mechanism is uncertain, but *in vivo* gold undoubtedly alters the properties of collagen.

Kinetics
Rapidly absorbed after i.m. injection and extensively bound to plasma proteins. Weekly injections are sufficient to maintain constant plasma levels.

Toxicity
Reactions most commonly occur during the initial course of injections.
1   Dermatitis − any degree from itching to severe exfoliative dermatitis may occur.
2   Renal damage − the appearance of albuminuria may signal renal tubular damage. Severe nephrosis can occur.
3   Blood dyscrasias − thrombocytopenia and more rarely aplastic anaemia.

CORTICOSTEROIDS

There are four types of hormonal steroid: anabolic steroids, sex steroids, mineralocorticoids and glucocorticoids.

Steroid drugs are natural or synthetic congeners of the glucocorticoid steroids normally secreted by the adrenal glands.

The natural production of glucocorticoids is stimulated by ACTH (Adrenocorticotrophic hormone) which is secreted by the pituitary gland. ACTH is itself released by a hormone from the hypothalamus. The hypothalamic-pituitary-adrenal (HPA) axis is subject both to central control and to the negative influence of plasma glucocorticoid levels; as the plasma cortisol level rises the activity of the H-P-A axis falls accordingly. The response to large doses of steroid drugs given over a long period of time, is total H-P A axis shutdown.

Hydrocortisone is the parent drug and occurs naturally; it has predominantly glucocorticoid but also some mineralocorticoid (sodium retaining) activity. Synthetic congeners have been developed which are more potent than hydrocortisone and lack the sodium-retaining action. A

major advance has been the 9a-fluorosubstituted compounds whose
advantages are shown in Table 4.3.

Table 4.3

Preparation	Tablet size mg	Anti-inflamm. effect	Sodium retaining effect
Hydrocortisone	20	1	1
Prednisolone	5	5	0.8
Betamethasone (9a-fluoro-)	0.5	40	0

Pharmacological actions of glucocorticoids (prolonged administration)

1 Anti-inflammatory (potent). An anti-inflammatory action is obtained
only in doses which greatly exceed the physiological requirements of the
body, and at such doses serious unwanted effects are inevitable.
2 Sodium metabolism (weak). Hydrocortisone and prednisolone have a
weak sodium retaining effect; with other synthetic analogues it is
virtually nil.
3 Carbohydrate metabolism. Insulin is antagonised and conversion of
liver glycogen to glucose is increased; the result may be hyperglycaemia
and glycosuria. Corticosteroids will disturb diabetic control.
4 Protein metabolism. Protein breakdown is encouraged. The results
are muscle-wasting, osteoporosis (loss of bone matrix), capillary fragility
(bruising) and poor wound healing.
5 Fat metabolism. Fat is deposited centrally — in the face, shoulders,
and trunk (Cushingoid appearance).
6 Behaviour. The personality may become euphoric (sometimes
depressed) and hallucinations can occur.
7 Growth failure. Children on long-term steroids may put on weight
through excessive deposition of fat but fail to grow normally.

Uses

Glucocorticoids and Synthenic congeners have three main uses:
1 The treatment of inflammation.
2 Substitution therapy (p.133).
3 Treatment of shock.
  Acute adrenal insufficiency resulting either from sudden withdrawal of
pharmacological doses or from overwhelming stress during substitution
therapy (Addisonian Crisis) will require treatment with large doses of
corticosteroid (for details see p. 160).

Treatment of inflammation

Formulations of anti-inflammatory glucocorticoids are available to treat a wide variety of inflammations whether systemic, intra-articular or topical. The uses and indications for steroid therapy are major and often controversial topics in therapeutics. Most of the detailed discussion lies outwith the scope of this book, but some basic principles apply when systemic steroid therapy is contemplated.

1   A single dose or short (i.e. 72-hour) course of corticosteroids in the absence of contra-indicatons may be considered harmless even at high dosage.
2   The longer the course of therapy, the greater the chance of serious toxicity.
3   The decision to use long-term steroids must not be taken lightly; although the initial therapeutic benefit may be immense, the commitment (particularly on the part of the patient) to continue the drugs may be lifelong.
4   In long-term therapy the optimum dose is the minimum which offers acceptable therapeutic effect.
5   The dose must be continually reviewed as the diseases under treatment commonly undergo natural fluctuations in intensity.
6   The anti-inflammatory action of steroids is in no way curative.
7   The sudden withdrawal of therapeutic doses of steroids may precipitate an adrenal crisis; withdrawal should always be gradual and stepwise over at least 10-14 days.
8   Whether steroids are being prescribed for physiological or therapeutic reasons, the dosage regime must be flexible and may require to be increased many fold in anticipation of or during stress (see below).

Hydrocortisone

Presentation
Tablets 10 mg, 20 mg
Lozenges 2.5 mg
Injection i.m. or i.v.
   Acetate: Vial 125 mg in 5 ml
   Sodium phosphate: Vial 100 mg in 1ml
   Sodium succinate: Vial 100 mg 500 mg powder.
   Also available as cream; ointment (with tetracycline neomycin), and lotion.

Administration

For dermatoses and 'cold sores' a 1 % hydrocortisone cream or ointment is applied twice daily. In the treatment of systemic inflammation and collagen disease, prednisolone is usually preferred. In the emergency treatment of asthma, hydrocortisone 100 mg-400 mg (depending upon response) is given by i.v. injection or infusion.

Hydrocortisone is given by i.v. injection to "steroid" patients in situations of abnormal stress, e.g. surgery or sudden trauma such as a traffic accident.

Betamethasone, Dexamethasone and Triamcinolone:

Potent anti-inflammatory glucocorticoids which have virtually no sodium retaining action. Betamethasone is widely used as a topical application to mucosa, skin and eyes, triamcinolone is available as a dental paste in carboxymethyl-cellulose.

Toxicity of steroid drugs
The conflict facing the practitioner contemplating the use of cortico-steroids lies between the immediacy of symptom relief, always appreciated by the patient, and the long delay in appearance of toxic effects which must be appreciated by the prescriber. The problem does not apply to the short-term use of steroids in dermatitis, acute asthma and oral ulceration, but the dental practitioner should be familiar with the hazards of long-term steroid therapy, particularly in relation to poor tissue healing, exposure to infection and increased dosage requirements before, during and after surgery (see below).

Even assuming that systemic steroids have been prescribed correctly and rationally, it is virtually impossible for the patient to escape some long-term toxicity if the dose exceeds 7.5 mg prednisolone (or equivalent) daily.

Admitting then the inevitability of toxicity, the prescriber must be certain that the toxic effects over 10-15 years are outweighed by the therapeutic advantages over the same period; a 'well now – pay later' approach is not justified. The following are the more important toxic effects which appear clinically; they refer to patients on pharmacological, not physiological (i.e. substitution) doses of glucocorticoids.

1 Exaggeration of physiological action; i.e. diabetes, hypertension, fluid retention and muscular weakness.
2 Impaired tissue healing.
3 Exposure to infection – the absence of inflammatory responses to chronic infections such as TB may render them clinically undetected for long periods.

4   Retardation of growth in children; this may be serious and is a constant accompaniment of long-term therapy.

5   Osteoporosis, particulary in old age and commonly leading to vertebral collapse.

6   Gastric ulceration, haemorrhage and even perforation.

7   Cataracts.

8   Renal stones (hypercalciuria).

9   Adrenal suppression: whether on physiological or pharmacological doses, the patient has no endogenous production of glucocorticoid.

Prevention of Adrenal crisis
Prior to a major dental procedure, the "steroid" patient should receive 100-200 mg (depending on body size) hydrocortisone i.m. If prolonged surgery is contemplated an i.v. infusion of 5 % dextrose should be set up containing 500 mg hydrocortisone; hypotension is the first sign of impending cardiovascular collapse. Hydrocortisone 100 mg should be given following the procedure (orally unless general anaesthetic used). Oral hydrocortisone or prednisolone should be given 6-hourly in decreasing dosage during the convalescent period. These precautions should be observed up to one year following the withdrawal of therapeutic doses of steroids.

Treatment of Adrenal crisis
The immediate needs are water, salt, glucose and hydrocortisone. Salt and water are given as an isotonic sodium chloride infusion to which can be added glucose, 5-10 %. Hydrocortisone 100 mg should be given i.v. immediately followed by 100 mg 6-8 hourly via the i.v. infusion. The precipitating cause should be sought and corrected.

ACTH (adrenocorticotrophic hormone)

ACTH is released from the anterior pituitary gland under the influence of a hypothalamic releasing factor. It is a polypeptide hormone which stimulates the adrenal cortex. Synthetic ACTH is sometimes used medically in place of pharmacological doses of corticosteroids.

Pharmacological actions
1   Release of adrenal steroids: principally hydrocortisone but to a lesser extent anabolic steroids. Aldosterone (mineralocorticoid) is not under ACTH control.

2   Large doses of ACTH may cause the hyperpigmentation also seen in Addison's disease (primary adrenal failure in which ACTH levels are high).

Kinetics
Not absorbed orally (proteolytic breakdown), and may only be administered by injection.

Toxicity
1   Almost entirely related to the pharmacological quantities of adreno-cortical steroids produced under its influence.
2   Rare hypersensitivity reactions.

Antihistamines

Histamine effects can be blocked in three ways:
1   By prevention of histamine release: corticosteroids and sodium cromoglycate (p.84) block different stages of the hypersensitivity reaction described on p.152.
2   Competitive antagonism (histamine receptor blockade) — these antagonists are the true antihistamines discussed below.
3   Physiological antagonism: adrenaline opposes the broncho-constrictor and peripheral vasodilator actions of histamine.
   Antihistamines are a heterogenous group all of which have a variety of other pharmacological actions, principally sedation; no *selective* histamine blocker has yet been developed.

Pharmacological actions of antihistamines
1   Competitive antagonism of histamine or H_1 receptors (i.e. exclude gastric secretion).
2   Sedation — antihistamines can reduce agitation, induce sleep, reduce vertigo and related nausea. Even in small doses cognitive performance may deteriorate and reaction time lengthen.
3   Anti-Parkinsonian effect — rigidity may improve.

Kinetics
Well-absorbed orally; can be administered parenterally.

Toxicity
Dizziness, fatigue and sedation are the commonest. Patients taking anti-histamines should not be allowed to drive private or public transport vehicles or work near exposed machinery. Atropinic effects can occur, such as dry mouth.

Promethazine

Presentation
Tablets sugar coated 10 mg, 25 mg

Elixir 5 mg in 5 ml
Injection 25 mg/ml
Cream 28 W/V.

Administration
As an anti-inflammatory drug it is applied to the following situations:
1   Acute urticaria — parenteral injection 25-50 mg for rapid effect.
2   Angioneurotic oedema; this may be life-threatening and adrenaline,
0.2 ml 1:1000 solution s.c. has a more rapid effect.
Antihistamines, if used, should be given i.m.
3   Seasonal hay-fever. Dose 10 mg q.i.d. Asthma responds poorly.
4   Pruritus (generalized pruritus is an important symptom of many
systemic diseases; its cause should always be sought). (May be found in
combination with ipecacuanha and quaiac, or coedeine and ephedrine as
cough expectorant and suppressant respectively).

Alternative drug
Chlorpheniramine.

4.15   DEPRESSION

Tricyclic antidepressants
   Imipramine
   Amitryptiline
   Nortryptiline
   Protryptiline
   Doxepin
MAO Inhibitors
   Phenelzine
Amphetamines
   Dextroamphetamine
Lithium carbonate
   Corticosteroids

THE ANTIDEPRESSANT DRUGS IN PERSPECTIVE

The advent of safe and effective antidepressant drug therapy came with
the introduction of tricyclic drugs following a fortuitous observation of
their antidepressant effect by Kuhn in 1958.

   This group of drugs has been a major therapeutic discovery and ranks in
importance with that of the antibiotics. Up to 80 % of psychotically
depressed patients respond to tricyclic drugs of the imipramine type. As a
result, depression is no longer confined to the area of specialist pyschiatry;
with care it can be treated in the general practitioner's surgery with

minimal disturbance of the patient's environment.

Depression appears to be an increasingly common symptom of modern living and has assumed the proportions of a major medical problem.

PHYSIOLOGY OF DEPRESSION

Reactive depression is usually considered to be an extension of normal human experience (such as excessive grief); it is resistant to anti-depressant drugs and tends to resolve spontaneously with time.

Endogenous depression is not primarily related to environmental change; it not only involves a change of mood but also somatic function such as sleep pattern, appetite, concentration, bowel habit, etc.

At a cellular level, endogenous depression can be related to changes in sodium metabolism. During attacks there is a measurable failure of cells to extrude sodium through the membrane's "Sodium pump"; during recovery from an attack the intracellular sodium levels can be shown to fall towards normal. Electro-convulsive therapy (ECT) improves the cerebral sodium transfer rate in all those responsive to therapy, whereas the clinically unresponsive show no such change. All effective antidepressant drugs affect sodium transfer directly or indirectly.

INDIVIDUAL DRUGS

Tricyclic antidepressants (dibenzazepines)

Pharmacological actions
1   Antidepressant action: Adrenaline and nor-adrenaline stimulate the extrusion of sodium at the cell membrane while reducing cellular sodium uptake. Tricyclic antidepressants block the entry of nor-adrenaline into cells, resulting in its accumulation and intense activity around them; the effect is greatest in brain cells.
2   Anticholinergic effects: (similar to those of atropine, p.95); these may be important clinically.
3   Strong sedative action. (In some cases only).

Kinetics
Well absorbed orally and metabolized by the liver. A response may not be noticeable for many days but is achieved in 80 % of cases.

Toxicity
1   Anticholinergic effects: dry mouth, dilated pupils (blurring of vision) and tachycardia are the commonest atropinic effects. Cardiac dysrhythmias on therapeutic dosage may occur in those predisposed.

Sudden unaccountable death due to cardiac standstill has been reported in relation to tricyclics. Glaucoma and prostatic obstruction may be worsened.

2 Psychological effects: impairment of concentration and cognitive processes is common. Hallucination and excitement may occur.

3 Drug interactions:

  (a) Catecholamines: tricyclic drugs potentiate the action of catecholamines. The administration of even small amounts of adrenaline (as in local anaesthetic preparations) may precipitate serious rises in blood pressure and pulse rate.

  (b) Post-ganglionic adrenergic neurone blockers: guanethidine, bethanidine and debrisoquine (p.74) used in the treatment of hypertension are concentrated in adrenergic nerve endings by the same pump that normally takes up circulating catecholamines. Tricyclic antidepressants inhibit this pump (see above). The administration of imipramine to a patient already on guanethidine blocks and action of the latter and causes a rise in circulating catecholamines; the result is an unexpected rise rather than the anticipated fall in B.P.

  (c) MAO Inhibitors: Monoamine oxidase inhibitors are anti-depressant drugs which act by preventing the breakdown of catecholamines in the CNS. Their combination with tricyclics can result in excitement and a syndrome similar to that of atropine toxicity: tachycardia, tachyarrhythmias, hallucination and hyperreflexia.

Monoamine Oxidase Inhibitors (MAOI)

Pharmacological actions:

1 Central. This group prevents the breakdown of amines within the brain and encourages the extrusion of intracellular sodium. Large amounts of nor-adrenaline are stored, unmetabolized, in nerve endings.

2 Peripheral. The action is complex. A rise or fall in blood pressure may result. There should nowadays be little or no clinical indication for this group of drugs; only the important drug interactions will be considered further.

  (a) Drug potentiation: morphine, pethidine, phenothiazines, barbiturates.

  (b) Hypertensive crises. Drugs which liberate nor-adrenaline from nerve endings may cause hypertensive crises in those taking MAO Inhibitors because of the large amounts of nor-adrenaline stored (see above). Two such substances are commonly encountered.

· Phenylpropanolamine is commonly found in proprietary cold cures.
· Tyramine is contained in many foods. Cheese, broad beans, meat extracts, (sometimes given to patients with inter-maxillary fixation) and

chianti-type red wines *must* be avoided in those taking MAO Inhibitors.

Note
Injected adrenaline, which is broken down by plasma O-methyl transferase rather than neuronal monoamine oxidase, does not carry the risk of interaction with MAOI.

Amphetamines

Pharmacological actions
Sympathomimetic actions similar to those of adrenaline, accounting for (a) elevation of mood as a central effect and (b) α and β sympathetic effects. In addition, amphetamines result in *temporary* alertness, increased capacity to concentrate, and delayed onset of fatigue. They are marked appetite suppressants. Amphetamines induce dependence.

Toxicity
Principally habituation (see p.211). Acute toxicity may result in hallucinaion and convulsion. (The danger of amphetamines to athletes has been well documented; hyperpyrexia can occur on exercise followed by vascular collapse and death).

Lithium

Pharmacological actions
Lithium can substitute for sodium in extracellular fluid and in the depolarization of nerve cells. Once it occupies an intracellular position (i.e. following depolarization), it cannot be extruded by the "sodium pump", with the result that sodium itself tends to remain outwith the cell and intracellular levels remain low.

   Goitregenic in prolonged dosage.

Corticosteroids (p.156)

Mood is closely related to blood cortisol level. The administration of corticosteroids is often associated with euphoria, and depletion (i.e. Addison's disease) with depression. Direct measurement has shown that adrenocortical insufficiency limits the extrusion of sodium from the cell and is associated with a rise in cerebral intracellular sodium concentration.

   Steroids are not employed therapeutically as anti-depressants but the action may be a bonus to their use in distressing disease states.

4.16   INSOMNIA AND ANXIETY

Benzodiazepines
   Diazepam
   Nitrazepam
   Chlordiazepoxide
   Oxazepam
   Medazepam
Chloral derivatives
   Triclofos
   Dichloralphenazone
Phenothiazines
   Chlorpromazine
   Trifluoperazine
   Thioridazine
Barbiturates
   Phenobarbitone
   Amylobarbitone
   Pentobarbitone

THE PLACE OF DRUG THERAPY IN INSOMNIA AND ANXIETY

Acute anxiety is usually best treated by exploring and removing the cause. Chronic anxiety, especially when associated with depression, can respond usefully to drug therapy.

The role of drugs in chronic sleeplessness is less certain and the disruption of the sleep pattern in chronic anxiety is arguably a natural compensatory response. In any event two facts remain outstanding:
1   sleep requirements vary enormously among individuals, and
2   hypnotics do not induce natural sleep.

Tolerance and habituation commonly accompany the chronic usage of hypnotics; it may take many weeks to restore a normal sleep pattern following the withdrawal of a long-term hypnotic.

The readiness of doctors to prescribe hypnotics on demand, the difficulties of hypnotic withdrawal and the common assumption that loss of sleep indicates therapeutic intervention would together suggest that hypnotics are prescribed far too frequently.

SLEEP PATTERNS

Sleep is not simply a negative state of arousal; it is a period during which specific and intense physiological activity occurs. Health, both of mind and body, depends far more on the quality of sleep than its duration.

Normal sleep has two main phases, orthodox and paradoxical, which alternate. The onset of natural sleep is influenced mainly by the circadian rhythm of the body (biological time-clock) and such environmental factors as warmth, physical comfort, and monotony.

Orthodox sleep

Characterized by slow-wave electroencephalogram activity and lack of eye-movement. The pituitary gland, relatively quiescent during wakefulness, releases large amounts of growth hormone and prolactin during orthodox sleep. Growth hormone stimulates the synthesis of protein and nuclear acids; its release does not occur during light sleep or during nocturnal rest which is lacking in sleep. Whether natural restorative processes are significantly affected is unknown.

Paradoxical sleep

A period of orthodox sleep is followed by a short period (20-30 min) of paradoxical sleep during which cerebral blood-flow is even higher than during waking hours; EEG activity is intense. Rapid eye movments (REM) and dreaming characterize this phase. There is no evidence that loss of dreaming, through interruption of the paradoxical phase, engenders emotional disturbance.

INSOMNIA AND ANXIETY

Anxiety may be related to insomnia in two ways:

1   It may be the cause; stress anxiety is becoming increasingly symptomatic of modern living.

2   It may also be the result. There is a wide variation in sleep requirements and some believe themselves insomniacs only because they fail to sleep the 'normal' eight hours.

Anxiety commonly results from emotional conflict. Reasons for the conflict may be readily identifiable in terms of worry or stress or may be wholly unaccountable. The emotional reaction may lead to depression (anxiety-depression), introspection and social isolation. The physical signs of anxiety result from an associated increase in sympathetic outflow from the hypothalamus. The typical signs are tremor, mydriasis, tachycardia and sweating (cf thyrotoxicosis). Patterns of sleep, eating and bowel action are commonly likewise disturbed.

APPLICATION OF DRUGS TO INSOMNIA AND ANXIETY

In general, the only difference between anxiolytic (or sedative) drugs and hypnotics is one of dosage; any sedative is hypnotic in large dosage and likewise a hypnotic in lesser dosage may be a useful sedative.

INSOMNIA

Very little is known of the physiological disturbances which may result from the use of hypnotic drugs. Benzodiazepines are known to abolish the EEG slow-wave activity of orthodox sleep and barbiturates reduce the duration and intensity of paradoxical sleep. The tricyclic antidepressants abolish REM.

Of possibly greater importance are rebound phenomena affecting sleep. Alcohol and barbiturates taken at night induce deep sleep initially but towards morning sleep becomes broken and restless, inciting the "insomniac" to take more of the drug the following night. Such cumulative effects are often mitigated by tolerance which is partly metabolic, on the part of the liver, and partly physiological, on the part of the brain. The changes in the brain tend to oppose the desired actions of the drug. If the hypnotic is suddenly withdrawn the effects of tolerance become unmasked; increased anxiety, restlessness, bizarre dreaming and REM sleep result.

ANXIETY

There are three rather indistinct groups of drugs:
1   *Anxiolytics*, claimed to be more specific with less tendency to sedate. Alternative term: minor tranquillizers. The best examples are members of the benzodiazepine group.
2   *Tranquillizers*, alternatively major tranquillizers or neuroleptics. These comprise phenothiazines and antihistamines. Their action (according to dose) may be to induce sedation, reduce aggression, anxiety and the cerebral response to vestibular disturbances such as occur in vertigo and motion sickness (p.104).
3   *Sedatives*. Drugs such as barbiturates are primarily sedative in action and produce more sleepiness in relation to their anxiety-reducing property than do the anxiolytics or major tranquillizers.

SPECIFIC DRUG GROUPS

Benzodiazepines (diazepam is frequently used in dentistry)

Pharmacological actions
Anxiolytic in small doses.
Hypnotic in larger doses.

Amnesia. In high serum concentrations (achieved by i.v. injection) benzodiazepines have a valuable anaesthetic and amnestic action (p.51).
Anticonvulsant.
Muscle relaxant (central action).

Kinetics
All are well absorbed orally.

Toxicity
Generally trivial. "Hangover" effects may occur in hypnotic doses. Plasma phenytoin (anticonvulsant) levels may rise in combination with benzodiazepines.
   Note: Fatal overdose is virtually unknown even with massive doses (i.e. 80 tablets).

Chloral derivatives

Pharmacological actions
Exclusively sedative/hypnotic. Frequently used in the very young and very old because of its safe and predictable action.

Kinetics
Well absorbed orally.

Toxicity
Interactions with:
· Alcohol. The drugs are mutually potentiating.
· Warfarin. Chloral metabolites displace warfarin from protein-binding sites (p.174) increasing its free plasma concentration. At the same time enzyme induction may occur which tends to reduce warfarin concentrations.

Phenothiazines

The parent drug is chlorpromazine which has a global action on behavioural and emotional state.

Pharmacological actions
Reduces agitation and aggression in doses which do not significantly impair consciousness.
Produce a state of physical lethargy and emotional indifference.
Anti-emetic.
Muscle-relaxant (central action).

Potentiates the action of all CNS depressants including analgesics (useful), alcohol and anaesthetics.
a-adrenoceptor blocking effect (hypotensive).

Kinetics
Well absorbed from the G.I. tract (irritant on i.m. injection). Therapeutic effects may last several months following withdrawal. It is metabolized by the liver.

Toxicity
1   Dystonic reactions and Parkinsonian-like syndrome (usually only after long-term administration).
2   Jaundice (allergic cholestasis) in about 1 % patients.
3   Blood dyscrasias.
4   Postural hypotension.
5   Rashes.

Related Drugs
Promazine. More sedative, less hepatotoxic and safer in the elderly.
   Trifluoperazine. Relatively stimulant, less hepatoxic and particularly liable to produce severe dystonic reactions.
   Thioridazine. Less liable to produce unwanted effects in the elderly.

Barbiturates

A group of drugs which differ mainly in the intensity of hypnosis they induce. Apart from the rapidly acting barbiturate anaesthetics (p.45) any one of the barbiturates produces an effect lasting about 8 hr; the traditional classification into short, medium and long-acting barbiturates relates to plasma $t\frac{1}{2}$ and not to therapeutic effect.

Pharmacological actions
Sedative, hypnotic or anaesthetic according to dose.
Anticonvulsant (phenobarbitone only).

Kinetics
All hypnotic/sedative barbiturates are well absorbed orally. Phenobarbitone in daily doses becomes cumulative. Barbiturates are metabolised by liver enzymes and their metabolism becomes self-induced so that the plasma $t\frac{1}{2}$ of the barbiturate (and many other drugs) becomes shortened with time: this is one aspect of barbiturate tolerance.

Toxicity
1   Undue drowsiness when used as an anxiolytic.

2 Drug interactions: these are due to enzyme induction in the liver, affecting principally phenytoin (with which it is commonly used as an anticonvulsant) and warfarin, resulting in a fall in their blood levels. Conversely the sudden withdrawal of barbiturates when used in combination with either warfarin or phenytoin may result in a significant rise in their plasma levels.

3 Dependence (p.207).

4 Porphyria in those predisposed.

5 Paradoxical arousal in the elderly.

6 Coma, respiratory and sometimes fatal cardiovascular depression in overdose.

4.17 THROMBO-EMBOLISM AND HEREDITARY HAEMORRHAGIC DISORDERS

Anticoagulants
    Oral anticoagulants: Phenindione, Warfarin
    Heparin
Anticoagulant antagonists (Antidotes)
    Vitamin K
    Protamine sulphate
Fibrinolytic drugs
    Streptokinase
Anti-plasmin drugs
    Epsilon aminocaproic acid
Clotting factors
    Anti-haemophilic globulin (AHG, Factor VIII)
    Christmas factor (Factor IX)

PATHOPHYSIOLOGY

The consistency of normal blood is maintained by an equilibrium between a tendency to form clot (thrombosis) and a tendency to dissolve clot (fibrinolysis). The thrombotic and fibrinolytic systems in blood are in constant *dynamic* balance so that disturbances in blood clotting are the result of dynamic changes (e.g. acceleration or deceleration) in one or other opposing force:

	Thrombin	
Thrombosis	⟵———————	Fibrinolysis
(clot formation)	———————⟶	(clot lysis)
	Plasmin	

Disturbances in clot formation

Thrombosis usually arises as a result of:
1   tissue damage where it normally serves a protective function; or
2   blood stasis.
    Certain drugs (e.g. oestrogen) may also induce thrombosis.
    Blood-clotting is a natural and essential protection against blood loss
following trauma. Damaged tissue initiates a series of chemical and
physical reactions which push the above equilibrium to the left. The
reactions involve plasma globulins known as clotting factors; the end-
product is thrombin which causes fibrinogen in the blood to polymerize
into strands of fibrin which contract and seal the wound.
    Stasis is an unnatural phenomenon; it results from obstruction to blood
flow. Commonly this is due to venous incompetence (e.g. varicosis) or to
local pressure on veins (e.g. during prolonged general anaesthesia). Damage
to platelets and vessel wall during stasis initiates a clotting process resulting
in thrombosis within the vessel lumen.
    The above remarks are directed primarily at venous thrombosis.
Coronary artery thrombosis is commoner but its pathogenesis is ill-
understood and therapeutic efforts at prevention are singularly ineffective.
    Clotting factor *deficiencies* are usually congenital and result in excess
blood loss after trauma and in the severest cases spontaneous bleeding
through unopposed fibrinolysis.

Disturbances in clot lysis

Plasmin is a fibrinolysin constantly being formed from plasminogen in the
blood stream. Excessive trauma, infection with fibrinolysin-(streptokinase-)
producing streptococci, and certain disease states (e.g. prostatic carcinoma)
may accelerate fibrinolytic activity. When natural or pathological blood
clots are formed natural fibrinolysins respond by slowly dissolving the
thrombus; the process may take days or weeks in the case of a large
thrombus.

APPLICATION OF DRUGS TO ABNORMALITIES OF
BLOOD-CLOTTING

A tendency to thrombosis may result from accelerated thrombin activity
or (rarely) from reduced fibrinolysis. Similarly a tendency to bleed may be
the result of reduced thrombin activity or accelerated fibrinolysis.
    Drugs are aimed at restoring the clotting equilibrium when it is
threatened or disrupted by disease states.
    Drug therapy in such situations demands fine control.

GENERAL PRINCIPLES

1 Always question for bleeding tendency in the clinical history.
2 Prescribe drugs with great caution for patients taking oral anticoagulants.
3 Consultation with the Regional Haemophilia Centre is mandatory when dental surgery is contemplated in haemophiliacs or patients with similar haemorrhagic disorders.

Thrombosis

Anticoagulants are used to prevent thrombosis and fibrinolytic drugs to dissolve clots once formed.

General indications

Anticoagulants
1 Deep venous thrombosis and pulmonary embolism (to prevent further thrombosis).
2 Mitral valve disease with atrial fibrillation (stasis occurs in the enlarged chambers of the fibrillating atria, resulting in development of thrombus).
3 Arterial thrombosis (to prevent extension of thrombus).
4 Myocardial infarction. The rationale is prevention of venous thromboembolism in poor risk patients (e.g. those confined to prolonged bed-rest, those with a previous history of venous thrombosis and those suffering the complications of infarction: shock, heart failure and dysrhythmias).

Fibrinolytic drugs
1 Venous thrombosis and pulmonary embolism.
2 Arterial thrombosis. Success with fibrinolytic drugs often depends upon accessibility and accurate localization of the thrombus.

DRUGS WHICH REDUCE THROMBIN ACTIVITY
(anticoagulants)

Anticoagulant drugs reduce clotting factor production or block the final reaction of thrombin and fibrinogen.

Phenindione (Indanedione group)

Pharmacological action
Prevents formation of clotting factors by liver.

Kinetics
Absorbed orally. Largely bound to plasma proteins and metabolized by liver enzymes.

Toxicity
May cause allergy in the form of skin rash or blood dyscrasia.

Warfarin (Coumarin group)

Pharmacological action
Similar to phenindione.

Kinetics
Absorbed orally. Strongly bound to plasma proteins and metabolized by non-specific liver enzymes.

Toxicity
Extremely rare.

Drug interactions
Warfarin is strongly protein-bound and is subject to displacement by such drugs as phenylbutazone, phenytoin and sulphonylureas. Its plasma level may be lowered by drugs which induce liver enzymes (e.g. barbiturates, alcohol).

Heparin

Pharmacological action
Principally physical antagonism to the action of thrombin. It interferes little with blood clotting factors and occurs naturally in most cells.

Kinetics
Only active by injection. The maximum effect is immediate and rapidly wears off within 4-6 hours. It is excreted by liver and kidney.

Toxicity
Alopecia (hair loss) is an occasional adverse effect, though transient.

ANTAGONISTS

The action of heparin may be reversed immediately by protamine. Warfarin and phenindione effects may be reversed by Vitamin K but a delay of up to 12 hours (during which normal levels of clotting factors are restored) is inevitable.

Laboratory control of anticoagulant therapy

Test	Prothrombin time	Thrombotest	Whole Blood Clotting time
Normal blood	10 - 14 secs.	100 %	5 - 10 mins.
Oral anticoagulation	~2 x normal	5 - 15 %	–
Heparin anticoagulation	–	–	~2 x normal

DRUGS WHICH ACCELERATE FIBRINOLYSIS (fibrinolytics)

Streptokinase

Pharmacological action
A plasminogen activator which converts the inert plasminogen into plásmin. Plasmin accelerates clot dissolution.

Kinetics
Absorbed by buccal mucus membranes but usually given by i.v. infusion. Duration of action short.

ANTAGONISTS

Antiplasmins such as epsilon aminocaproic acid – EACA (see below).

Bleeding Tendency

DRUGS WHICH REDUCE FIBRINOLYTIC ACTIVITY

Hyperplasminaemic states due to excessive release of plasminogen activator (e.g. severe trauma, obstetrical haemorrhage) may result in a tendency to haemorrhage.

Epsilon aminocaproic acid (EACA)

Pharmacological action
Antiplasmin

Kinetics
Absorbed orally or by injection. Short half-life.

Toxicity
Its pharmacological action may be dangerous if given injudiciously.

Presentation
Syrup 200 mg/ml. Injection Vials 5 g in 50 mls.

Administration
Aminocaproic acid may be used as an antidote following an excessive
response to fibrinolytic drugs. It is used routinely during dental extraction
in haemophiliacs (see below).

Side-effects
Occasionally hypotension, nausea, abdominal discomfort and nasal congestion may occur. It should be avoided early in pregnancy.

DRUGS WHICH ACCELERATE THROMBIN ACTIVITY

Specific clotting factor deficiences are the cause of the hereditary
haemorrhagic diseases; they respond temporarily to plasma concentrates
containing the missing factor. Vitamin K is a precursor of many clotting
factors and it too may be deficient in malabsorption states or liver
disease, necessitating the therapeutic use of Vitamin K preparations.

Anti-haemophilic globulin (Factor VIII)

Pharmacological action
Replacement in deficiency disease (haemophilia).

Kinetics
Given by infusion of a suitable concentrate. Its maximal effect is
immediate and the half-life is short (8-12 hours). AHG is unstable in stored
blood.

Sources
Various blood products may be used as a source of AHG. Their relative
AHG content is:

Fresh blood	100 %
Stored blood	
(7 days old)	20 %
Fresh frozen plasma	80 %
Cryoprecipitate	100 % yield

AHG levels are measurable in the laboratory as a percentage of normal.
In severe haemophilia the levels may be zero, in milder cases as high as

20 %. The aim of treatment is to restore the circulating AHG to a coagulating level (about 30 %).

Note
Serum hepatitis is a potential problem whenever blood products are being used. Cryoprecipitate AHG is derived from pooled plasma which diminishes the risk of a high dose of virus by virtue of dilution.

Christmas factor (Factor IX)

Pharmacological action
Replacement in deficiency disease (Christmas disease).

Kinetics
Similar to AHG. Christmas factor, however is stable in stored blood for up to 14 days, and dried plasma retains substantial factor IX activity.

Vitamin K
Vitamin K is found naturally in the diet and is synthesized by gut bacteria.

Pharmacological action
An essential precursor for the manufacture of prothrombin and other clotting factors in the liver.

Kinetics
The natural vitamin (phytomenandione) is fat-soluble and given orally is only poorly absorbed in the absence of bile. Water-soluble analogues are not dependent on bile for absorption.

Toxicity
Phytomenandione is non-toxic. Water-soluble analogues may cause haemolysis.

CLINICAL MANAGEMENT OF HAEMORRHAGIC DISEASE

Haemophilia and Christmas disease are a major problem in dentistry, particularly if emergency dental treatment is required. The following principles should be observed.
1   Major procedures should be made elective so that the patient can be adequately prepared.

2   Dental extractions should not be undertaken without prior consultation with a specialist in haemorrhagic disease. 40 Haemophilia Centres are distributed throughout the British Isles and may be contacted by telephone day or night. Ideally major dental surgery should be conducted in such a Centre.

3   The correct diagnosis must be ascertained. Haemophilia and Christmas disease are very similar in presentation but are treated differently. Von Willebrand's disease (unfortunately also termed pseudo-haemophilia) is again similar in presentation but is due chiefly to an inherited capillary defect, although in some cases there is a Factor VIII deficiency.

4   Intramuscular injections must be avoided. Prolonged pressure should be applied following intravenous injections. Even local anaesthetic injections are not without risk and regional blocks are contra-indicated.

DENTAL EXTRACTION IN HAEMOPHILIACS

A typical regime (Rizza 1974) is as follows:

1   Morning of operation: transfusion of cryoprecipitate designed to raise the Factor VIII level to 50 % of normal, followed by an injection of E.A.C.A. in a dose of 0.1 g/Kg body weight.

2   Following extraction, oral E.A.C.A. 0.1 g/Kg every 6-10 hours for 7-10 days. No further cryoprecipitate is given unless the patient bleeds.

CHRISTMAS DISEASE

Factor IX

The same principles apply to the prevention and management of haemorrhage in Christmas disease as in haemophilia. However, Factor IX is more stable and stored blood or dried plasma may be used to arrest bleeding. The disease is milder than haemophilia. The danger of serum hepatitis exists in treatment.

VON WILLEBRAND'S DISEASE

There is no specific treatment. Corticosteroids are ineffective. Fresh blood is required if blood loss is acute; Factor VIII (AHG) may be helpful in some cases.

Local measures to arrest dental bleeding and protect the clot include suturing, dental *splints* and *topical application of thrombin*. The choice varies with the dental surgeon.

4.18 DRUGS USED IN MALIGNANCY

Cytotoxic Drugs
Alkylating agents
    Chlorambucil
    Melphalan
    Cyclophosphamide
    Mustine
    Busulphan
Antimetabolites
    Methotrexate
    Mercaptopurine
    Azathioprine
    Cytarabine
Antibiotics
    Bleomycin
    Daunorubicin
    Doxorubicin
Vinca alkaloids
    Vinblastine
    Vincristine
Nitrosoureas
    Carmustine
    Lomustine
Miscellaneous
    Procarbazine
    Dacarbazine

Hormones
Oestrogens
    Stilboestrol
Androgens
    Nandrolone (testosterone)
Progestogens
    Norethisterone

Enzymes
L-asparaginase

Corticosteroids
Prednisolone

INTRODUCTION

The successful treatment of malignant disease is a very recent advance in therapeutics. The major achievements have been made with the treatment of leukaemias and lymphomas. Carcinomas remain resistant to treatment although research in the area of immunotherapy shows signs of promise. There are three main approaches to the treatment of malignancy:

· Drugs (cytotoxic, hormonal, enzymatic)
· Radiation
· Surgical resection (for either the tumour or, if the tumour is hormone dependent, palliative resection of the appropriate endocrine gland).

The dentist is concerned not only with oral neoplasms but also with the oral complications of systemic malignancies. His role is vital in the early detection of oral malignancy and the dental team may be asked to construct a prosthesis following ablative surgery.

Our main concern is with cytotoxic drugs, which can predispose to infection and marrow dysfunction; either complication may be present with signs in the mouth or pharynx.

Reticuloses (leukaemias and lymphomas) can no longer be considered uniformly fatal. Aggressive and intensive chemotherapy, criticized by many on account of the attendant toxicity, is more than justified by the increasing yield of cures.

The chemotherapy of malignancy is a highly-specialized area of medicine; it is the larger centres with the greatest experience, which obtain the best results.

PATHOPHYSIOLOGY OF MALIGNANCY

Much of the rationale for the modern drug treatment of malignancy has arisen from detailed studies in cell kinetics. The most fruitful work has been done with malignancies of the marrow and reticulo-endothelial (R.E) system — diseases which are collectively termed the reticuloses.

Normal cells differentiate in an orderly fashion, perform their function for a reasonably constant period of time and are subsequently destroyed at a rate which matches their production. Transient upsets in this equilibrium are common (and protective) during infection. Reticuloses result from the aberrant behaviour of one cell or clone of cells which permanently and progressively upsets the equilibrium. This may be due to accelerated production or a fall in the rate of destruction; in many cases the aberrant cells fail to differentiate completely and excess numbers of functionless and variably immature cells are produced. Hence a leukaemia may be of the "stem-cell" type or "well-differentiated". In general, the less differentiated the cell type, the more malignant is the condition. The combined presence of excessive numbers of malfunctioning and lack of normal R.E. cells has three major effects:

· Infection; the body is deprived of its cellular defences.

· Marrow hypoplasia; normal marrow tissue is displaced by the invasion of non-functioning immature cells. The results are pallor (red cell deficiency), bleeding (platelet deficiency), and oral ulceration (white cell deficiency).
· Lymphoid tissue swelling — lymph nodes, spleen and liver swell with the excessive numbers of malignant cells.

SPECIFIC DRUG GROUPS

CYTOXIC DRUGS

These can be considered in groups according to their sites of action within the cell.
· Alkylating agents: act directly on the DNA system.
· Antimetabolites: act by competitive antagonism. They resemble structurally certain enzyme substrates within the cell and by combining with the appropriate enzymes, prevent further reaction.
· Antibiotics.
· Vinca (periwinkle) alkaloids.

HORMONES

Some tumours develop well in an environment where androgens predominate over oestrogens (carcinoma prostate) and vice versa (carcinoma breast). Therapeutic reversal of this favourable balance may lead to regression and control of the tumour over several years. Such a reversal may be achieved by drugs — oestrogens, androgens and progestogens, or by surgical resection of an appropriate endocrine gland — adrenalectomy, ovarectomy or pituitary ablation.

Adrenocorticosteroids have a direct cyto-reductive effect in lymphatic leukaemias and lymphosarcoma and also help to reduce immune haemolysis and thrombocytopenia which commonly accompany reticuloses.

ENZYMES

Asparaginase; some leukaemic cell-lines are dependent, as are all normal cells, on asparagine, yet unlike the latter are deficient in their ability to synthesize it. In the absence of adequate serum asparagine, the neoplastic cells die. Asparaginase destroys serum asparagine and selectively acts against the malignant cell. In practice, tolerance to this effect is rapidly gained by the malignant cell-line, so that asparaginase has had very limited usefulness so far.

IMMUNOTHERAPY

Recent evidence suggests that the immune response mounted by the body against tumour antigens becomes rapidly modified and ineffective. Non-specific immunizing procedures (i.e. with BCG vaccine) have been widely applied (empirically) to restore immune competence, but the problem of mounting an immune attack on tumour tissue has not been solved.

APPLICATION OF DRUGS TO RETICULOSES

All cellular chemistry is based upon reactions of DNA and RNA and most of the current chemotherapeutic drugs interfere with these processes at one stage or another. As might be expected, these drugs affect all cells, not just the malignant lines.

An important factor in the design of drug regimes is the differential in rates of multiplication between the malignant line of cells and the healthy lines. The greater the disparity, the easier it is to time "pulses" of therapy which "cripple" selectively the malignant cells. Although it is possible accurately to calculate multiplication rates of the different cell-lines in the individual, this approach has not proved any more successful in practice than applying empirical regimens. Most of the recent clinical research has been applied to evaluating different regimens in large numbers of patients with a single disease.

PRINCIPLES OF DRUG TREATMENT

· Malignant cells become resistant to drugs; the cyclical use of several drugs surmounts this problem.
· The efficacy of several drugs used in combination is additive; their specific toxicity may not be.
· The intermittent use of drugs may be more effective than daily administration. This is because the cell-doubling time of malignant cell-lines is commonly far *longer* than that of the normal cells. The rest period between doses allows the normal line to recover selectively.
· Acute leukaemias are treated in three phases, using different drug combinations in each:
Induction of remission
Consolidation (cyto-reduction)
Maintenance.
· Lymphomas are treated with repeated courses of a fixed combination of drugs, spaced at regular intervals with prolonged rest-periods between.

SPECIFIC CONDITIONS

ACUTE LEUKAEMIAS

Acute lymphoblastic

Predominantly a disease of childhood. Survival time is very closely related to success in inducing the first remission, nowadays achieved in about 90 % of patients with vincristine and prednisolone in combination. Further intensive chemotherapy, usually with courses of methotrexate, 6-mercaptopurine and cyclophosphamide given serially, achieves maximal reduction of the malignant cell population (consolidation). Methotrexate is commonly used for maintenance therapy. Should relapse occur, the regime must be repeated.

Acute myeloblastic

A disease affecting mainly adults and commonly a sequel to chronic myeloid leukaemia and polycythaemia rubra vera. The prognosis is poorer than that of acute lymphoblastic leukaemia.
Induction of remission: commonly cytarabine + daunorubicin. The drugs are given in repeated courses with 'rest' intervals between.
Consolidation: 6-mercaptopurine.
Maintenance: methotrexate.

CHRONIC LEUKAEMIAS

Chronic lymphatic

A disease of advancing years in which the milder form is benign and does not necessarily require treatment. Therapy, if indicated, is aimed at controlling the disease rather than obtaining radical cure.

Alkylating agents (chlorambucil, cyclophosphamide) are most successful and are given continuously. Local irradiation can successfully reduce the size of large glandular masses. Inter-current infection due to deficient immune responses are common on lymphatic leukaemia and should be treated vigorously (see below).

Chronic myeloid

One of a group of myeloproliferative diseases (polycythaemia vera, thrombocythaemia, myelofibrosis) which commonly overlap, with one cell-line predominating. The usual form of therapy is continuous busulphan (dose adjusted according to response) or occasionally intermittent radiotherapy with injected radioactive phosphorus P^{32}. When acute myeloblastic change supervenes, it should be treated accordingly (often with little success).

LYMPHOMAS

Hodgkin's disease (lymphoma)

The commonest of a number of related lymphoproliferative disorders. Localized disease of lymph nodes is treated by radiotherapy; chemotherapy is reserved for disseminated Hodgkin's disease.

Modern chemotherapy regimes use a combination of cytotoxic drugs which achieve not only an increasing number of cures but also induce remission more rapidly. A typical combination regime would include prednisolone, procarbazine, vinblastine and mustine hydrochloride (alkylating agent).

Myelomatosis

A malignant proliferation of plasma cells (immuno-competent lymphocytes). Chemotherapy is disappointing but some success has been obtained with the intermittent administration of prednisolone and an alkylating agent (melphalan or cyclophosphamide). Recently combination therapy with vincristine, melphalan and prednisolone has given encouraging results. A common symptom of myeloma is bone pain due to local invasion and this is best treated by local radiotherapy.

Other malignant diseases. Very few are currently amenable to chemotherapy.

COMPLICATIONS OF MALIGNANT DISEASE AMENABLE TO DRUG THERAPY

Anaemia
Hypoplastic anaemia is common in leukaemias and fresh blood transfusion if often indicated. Haemolytic anaemia due to red-cell antibodies is a feature of the lymphatic leukaemias and myelomatosis; corticosteroids (prednisolone) usually controls the haemolysis. Platelet destruction by antibodies may similarly respond.

Hypercalcaemia
Common in myelomatosis and responds to prednisolone.

Hyperuricaemia (gout)
Rapid nucleic acid turnover, a feature of reticuloses, results in high uric acid levels which may be controlled by allopurinal. Acute gout is best treated by phenylbutazone (in the absence of haemorrhagic tendency).

Renal failure
Leukaemias may terminate in renal failure. The prognosis of myelomatosis is closely related to renal function. Successful treatment of the primary disease prevents such complications.

Infection
Infection is both a complication of the malignant processes and of the chemotherapy used to treat them. In both cases there is a deficiency of immune response. Many malignancies are attended by toxic fevers and great care must be taken to differentiate those from infections which are liable to spread rapidly unless checked by specific antimicrobial drugs.

SIDE EFFECTS OF CHEMOTHERAPEUTIC DRUGS

Cytotoxic drugs damage all cells, affecting the most rapidly dividing cells (marrow, gut and skin) primarily. Generalized marrow hypoplasia is a constant complication of cytotoxic therapy; diarrhoea and skin ulceration are less common.

Infection is often opportunistic, the organisms being commensals of low virulence. Streptococcal throat infections, staphylococcal abscess and cellulitis are common. Superinfections with fungi such as monilia and aspergillus may be systemic or local to the mucous membranes or skinfolds. They must be identified and treated vigorously.

Local reactions: many cytotoxic drugs are seriously irritant and must be given by rapid i.v. infusion to avoid local tissue necrosis. Nausea and vomiting commonly attend such infusions and a phenothiazine anti-emetic (p.105) should be given beforehand.

Hormone treatment is attended by pharmacological effects. Long-term oestrogen therapy in the male may produce disfiguring and painful gynaecomastia in addition to fluid retention, and anabolic steroids in the female may have virilizing effects.

Radiotherapy may produce radiation burn, tissue necrosis and nausea in addition to marrow hypoplasia.

DENTAL CARE AND MALIGNANT DISEASE

The dentist is faced with problems of the malignancy itself and of the cytotoxic drugs or radiation used to treat it. The following principles should be observed, assuming that dental surgery is unavoidable.

· Major surgery should not be attempted without first consulting a specialist. He will be able to advise on the optimum time for operation and the best means of preparation.

· The major problems facing the dental surgeon are infection and bleeding. Haemorrhage due to serious platelet deficiency may be prevented if necessary by platelet infusions. Infection can be prevented by strict asepsis. Because simple and normally innocuous bacteria may produce virulent infections in immune deficiency states (e.g. lymphatic leukaemia, myeloma) "blind" antibiotic therapy is not justified and may cause serious confusion. If oral or systemic infection occurs after surgery, treatment must be preceded by attempts to culture the causative organism. Antibiotic prophylaxis is often advisable but remains a controversial matter. Only bactericidal drugs should normally be used.

· The precautions noted elsewhere (p.160) for those patients taking corticosteroid drugs must be rigidly observed.

· Whenever he is conducting an oral examination in a patient with malignancy, particularly reticulosis, the dentist should search carefully for signs of oral infection, particularly thrush, and of agranulocytosis (faucial ulceration). Herpes zoster is a common complication of the reticuloses.

4.19   EPILEPSY

Phenytoin
Phenobarbitone
Primidone
Troxidone
Sulthiame
Carbamazepine
Diazepam
Nitrazepam

GENERAL CONSIDERATIONS

Although most cases of epilepsy are idiopathic, the definable causes are numerous and some directly treatable. Even an isolated fit should be referred for full investigation. In established epilepsy there is sometimes a pattern (e.g. nocturnal fits only) and commonly precipitants (like alcohol) are known to the patient; it is important to recognise such patterns and avoid the precipitants.

The best choice of anticonvulsant drugs commonly results from trial and error. There are certain drugs best suited to a particular type of epilepsy but in general the choice is to be made from a few well-tried preparations.

4.19.2   PATHOPHYSIOLOGY

Numerous circumstances may give rise to a seizure focus. Acute foci may arise from fever (e.g. febrile convulsions of childhood) or local metabolic change due to changes in pH, electrolytes, or blood sugar content. Chronic (stable) foci commonly result from brain damage (often incurred at birth), from vascular changes, trauma or cerebral neoplasm. In the majority of cases the cause is unknown — idopathic epilepsy.

Nerve cells from an epileptic focus on the brain are excessively sensitive to stimulation. Such cells commonly show paroxysmal bursts of activity which correlate well with the EEG patterns characteristic of epilepsy. The *spread* of a paroxysm results in a seizure; the type of seizure depends on the origin of the paroxysm and on the pattern and extent of its spread. Once begun, the seizure is self-perpetuated by the recirculation of excitatory impulses. Spontaneous collapse of the "seizure loop" results in termination of the attack and is probably due to a rise in threshold potential and prolongation of refractory period of the cells involved. Inhibitory impulses from uninvolved cells also contribute. It is probable that "seizure cells" are pharmacologically different from their normal neighbours.

PATTERNS OF SEIZURE

The term 'epilepsy' (literally a seizure) denotes an alteration of consciousness. Convulsions may or may not accompany the seizure. The following patterns are common:

1   Grand mal (centrencephalic): characterized by total loss of consciousness and convulsions, clinically divisible into tonic and clonic phases.

2   Petit mal: brief attacks of altered consciousness, best described as absences but no convulsions. Common in childhood and may later develop into grand mal attacks.

3   Psychomotor (temporal lobe): Confused behaviour often accompanied by olfactory (smell) or gustatory (taste) hallucination.

Many other variants exist.

DRUGS AS A CAUSE OF EPILEPSY

Drugs may precipitate epilepsy, either directly or indirectly. The analeptic drugs (e.g. nikethamide) and other cerebral stimulants sometimes cause seizures; cerebral depressants may lead to anoxaemia and hypercapnia, both of which can be epileptogenic. Sudden withdrawal of the drugs used to control epilepsy may precipitate attacks. Commonly a combination of circumstances is the cause. Occasionally hyperventilation due to anxiety may lead to tetanic spasms, though consciousness is rarely altered.

DRUGS IN THE TREATMENT OF EPILEPSY

Anticonvulsant drugs act principally by stabilising normal cells, preventing spread from a discharging seizure focus. The possible physiological targets are threshold potential, synoptic transmission and refractory period.

Almost all anticonvulsant drugs are structurally similar to the parent compound phenobarbitone.

Phenytoin (diphenylhydantoin)

The most useful of the anticonvulsants.

Action

Prevents or reduces the spread of activity from a seizure focus, probably by blocking synaptic transmission. It has no sedative action on the brain, a fact of major therapeutic importance. (It also has specific cardiac antidys-rhythmic properties, p.95).

Kinetics

Well absorbed orally. The onset of action is slow and variable; a small minority of the population are exceedingly slow metabolizers of phenytoin. Therapeutic activity and toxicity correlate well with plasma concentrations of the drug which are nowadays frequently monitored to obtain optimum dosage. It is metabolized by liver microsomal enzymes; several drugs may interfere with the rate of breakdown:

· Phenobarbitone (commonly given with phenytoin) induces liver enzymes, yet simultaneously, competitively antagonizes the breakdown of phenytoin. The net result on plasma levels is unpredictable.

· Drugs which competitively inhibit phenytoin metabolism include Sulthiame (anticonvulsant) Isoniazid (anti-tubercular drug). The result is a rise in phenytoin plasma levels and unexpected toxicity may ensue.

Toxicity

Toxic effects may result from acute overdosage or from long-term administration.

· Acute overdosage. Oral overdosage disturbs mainly cerebellar and vestibular function, leading to ataxia, vertigo and nystagmus. These signs may also appear with cumulative toxicity.

· Chronic dosage. Gingival hyperplasia occurs in a minority of cases with pre-existing gingivitis. Edentulous gums are not affected.

· Folate deficiency leading to megaloblastic anaemia and occasionally peripheral neuropathy may occur after many years of treatment.

· Miscellaneous. Gastric upset, morbilliform skin-rash and blood dyscrasias sometimes occur. Jaundice has been reported. Teratogenesis (foetal malformation) is rare but demands strong indications before the drug is used in pregnancy.

Phenobarbitone

Action

All barbiturates are cerebral depressants but Phenobarbitone also has a specific anticonvulsant action. Like Phenytoin it raises the threshold of the motor cortex to aberrant electrical stimulation.

Kinetics

Well absorbed orally. About 25% is excreted unchanged in the urine. The remainder is metabolized by liver enzymes, which it strongly induces; the plasma *t½* of phenobarbitone therefore tends to fall progressively with chronic administration (tolerance) which may result in a loss of therapeutic effect unless the dose is appropriately increased.

Toxicity

· Occasional allergic reactions occur.
· Drug dependence can occur.
· Sudden withdrawal of phenobarbitone may lead to excitement, agitation and sometimes convulsion.
· The aged commonly respond to barbiturates with excitement rather than sedation.
· Barbiturate overdosage; the main effects are coma, respiratory and circulatory failure.

Alternative drugs

Primidone is similar to phenobarbitone.

Troxidone and ethosuxamide are frequently used in petit mal seizures.

Sulthiame is used principally to treat psychomotor (temporal lobe) seizures. It antagonizes the metabolism of phenytoin, more than doubling its blood level which may account for much of its therapeutic effect.

Carbamazepine is similar to phenytoin. It has a specific action in preventing the sensory nerve discharges which cause trigeminal and glosso-pharyngeal neuralgia.

Diazepam is a benzodiazepine drug with cerebral depressant action which is highly effective in continuous epileptic seizure (status epilepticus). Given i.v., its duration of action is short. Nitrazepam has proved effective in myoclonic spasm and hypsarrhythmia in children.

4.20   VITAMIN DEFICIENCY STATES

VITAMIN A
  Halibut Liver Oil BP.
Vitamins A and D BPC

VITAMIN B
  Vitamin B Tablets
  Vitamin B Compound Tablets BPC
VITAMIN C
  Ascorbic Acid
VITAMIN D
  Calcium with Vitamin D Capsules BP
  Calciferol Capsules strong BPC
  Vitamins A and D BPC
VITAMIN K
  Discussed on p.177

THE PHYSIOLOGICAL ROLE OF VITAMINS

Man is unable to synthesize his own supply of vitamins except for small amounts of cholecalciferol (Vitamin D_3) which are produced through the action of sunlight on a precursor in the skin. Sufficient vitamins are present in a well-balanced diet. Vitamin deficiency may be due to dietary lack, malabsorption, or to increased needs in the face of an otherwise adequate supply — e.g. pregnancy, lactation and the rapid growth of infancy.

Vitamins are trace substances vital to normal metabolism. Their function may be specific to a particular system; vitamin K is necessary for the synthesis of many blood-clotting factors, in particular prothrombin. B vitamins, on the other hand, are to be found in every cell as components of important enzyme systems.

Deficiency states are characterized by specific syndromes the study of which has led to a fuller understanding of the role that vitamins play. Vitamins are either fat soluble (A, D and K) or water soluble (B and C). Fat-soluble vitamins are only properly absorbed from the gut in the presence of adequate bile.

INDIVIDUAL VITAMINS

Vitamin A (Retinol)

Physiological action
A constituent of rhodopsin (visual purple), a light-sensitive pigment produced by the retina. It is claimed to have some pharmacotherapeutic value in hyperplastic skin conditions such as psoriasis.

Kinetics
Retinol is highly cumulative (mainly liver).

Toxicity
Those of over-dosage only. Acute toxicity may induce vomiting, drowsiness and even exfoliation. Chronic over-consumption can stimulate local bone growth (exostoses).

VITAMIN B COMPLEX

A group of unrelated substances originally thought to be a single dietary factor. The most important in terms of defined deficiency diseases are thiamine, pyridoxine and nicotinamide. Vitamin B complex deficiency is frequently associated with cheilitis and stomatitis. 'Pure' deficiency syndromes seldom occur.

Folic acid and cyanocobalamin (B_{12}) are haematinic substances discussed under 'Anaemia' (p.66).

Thiamine (B_1)

Deficiency syndrome: Beri-beri.

Physiological action
Thiamine is the coenzyme of carboxylase, itself an enzyme necessary for the metabolism of pyruvate and other keto-acids. A suspected deficiency of thiamine (e.g. in chronic alcoholism) may be demonstrated by measuring the patient's response to a measured dose of pyruvate (pyruvate tolerance test). Thiamine has no useful pharmacological actions and is non-toxic.

Pyridoxine (B_6)

Deficiency syndrome: mixed.

Physiological action
A coenzyme of transaminases required for the metabolism of protein and is distributed generally. Familial pyridoxine resistance has been described which responds to pharmacological doses.

Nicotinamide (B_2)

Deficiency syndrome: pellagra.

Physiological action
A constituent of co-dehydrogenases and vital to tissue oxidation processes. It is non-toxic.

Ascorbic Acid (Vitamin C)

Deficiency syndrome: scurvy.

Physiological action:
A strong reducing substance distributed generally. Appearances in scurvy
would suggest a specific role in maintaining the integrity of collagen tissue.
Pharmacological doses of ascorbic acid have the following effects, some of
which have established clinical values:
— Urinary acidification
— Reduction of incidence (doubtful) and severity (better evidence) of
common cold.
— Reduction of serum cholesterol (but may apply only to relatively
vitamin C-deficient populations).

Toxicity
Nil.

Vitamin D (see also p.132)

The collective name for a group of similar compounds. The principal
members are:
· Calciferol (D_2 plant origin).
· Cholecalciferol (D_3) animal origin.

Physiological action
High dosage simply results in high excretion. Lack of vitamin D does not
affect tooth calcification.
· Increases calcium absorption from the gut, tending to raise serum calcium
· Minor effect on renal tubules, promoting phosphage excretion.
· It has two effects on bone:
In rickets (and osteomalacia) and hypoparathyroidism it causes bone
deposition;
In healthy people it causes bone *resorption* and hypercalcaemia (also the
result of over-treating rickets with vitamin D).

Kinetics
Well absorbed orally in the presence of adequate bile (fat soluble vitamin).
It is metabolized in liver and kidney to pharmacologically more active
substances. Its optimal action in deficiency states may be delayed several
months and a large single injection may last 6-12 months. Its oral absorption is reduced by corticosteroid drugs. The drug is highly cumulative.

Toxicity
Excess of vitamin D leads to hypercalcaemia with attendant symptoms of

malaise, drowsiness, thirst and abdominal pain (sometimes peptic ulceration). Protracted hypercalcaemia leads to soft-tissue calcification; in particular renal calcification and subsequent renal failure.

Note
Vitamin D deficiency: rickets is still frequent among Asian immigrant populations in the UK.

THERAPEUTIC USE OF VITAMINS

The therapeutic use of vitamin preparations falls into four categories:
1   The treatment of overt deficiency syndromes (e.g. scurvy, rickets, osteomalacia). The cause of deficiency must first be sought.
2   Prevention of deficiency in certain well-recognised situations e.g. infants on powdered milk (A and D), total gastrectomy (B_{12}).
3   Pharmacological use of vitamins e.g. Vitamin C in the treatment of common cold (questionable), Vitamin D in hypoparathyroidism.
4   Treatment of 'malaise' or 'fatigue'. In 1971 1.6 % of all drugs prescribed by general practitioners were vitamin preparations (excluding the specific haemopoietic vitamins). The cost was £1.4 million. £80 million is spent yearly by the public on proprietary drugs sold over the counter, a substantial proportion of which are vitamins.
There is no evidence to suggest that vitamin deficiency is common in Britain but the public's belief in their efficacy and their strong placebo value are presumably the reasons behind such widespread use. Where genuine vitamin deficiency results from dietary deficiency or malabsorption, the syndromes which result are almost always mixed.

PART 5 · THE MANAGEMENT OF EMERGENCIES

5.1 SUGGESTED STOCK OF EMERGENCY DRUGS

Adrenaline 1: 1000 s.c. (ampoules 1 ml).
Hydrocortisone i.v. (ampoules 100 mg in 10 ml).
Aminophylline i.v. (ampoules 250 mg in 10 ml).
Promethazine i.v. (ampoules 25 mg in 1 ml).
500 ml dextrose or saline for i.v. infusion.
Oxygen (and Ambu-bag with face mask).

A set of endotracheal tubes and laryngoscopes (adult *and* paediatric sizes) should always be available, in addition to adequate suction apparatus.

5.2 ACUTE DRUG-INDUCED ANAPHYLAXIS

Definition

The response to a massive release into the circulation of histamine and similar vasoactive substances subsequent to an allergic reaction, and characterized by profound shock and bronchospasm.

Mechanism

The introduction of antigen into a suitably sensitized individual leads to antigen/antibody combination and the disintegration of connective tissue mast cells. The mast cell releases vasoactive substances whose pharmacological actions are:
Smooth muscle contraction
Vasodilatation of small vessels
Increase in capillary permeability

Presentation

Symptons occur within minutes of antigenic challenge. In dentistry the likeliest offenders are penicillin and local anaesthetics. Initially the patient may complain of generalized itching, abdominal colic and vomiting.

Bronchospasm with audible wheeze (acute asthma) soon follows. Laryngeal oedema may lead to stridor. The patient becomes rapidly pale or cyanosed, the blood pressure falls and he loses consciousness in a state of profound circulatory failure.

Prevention

A previous history of sensitivity to drugs must *always* be sought in *every* patient attending the dental surgery. Such sensitivity must be noted clearly on the patient's record card (preferably by coloured star or strip to attract attention) and of course the offending drug must be avoided at all costs. Patients known to be hypersensitive to particular drugs should ideally carry a metal bracelet to that effect.

Treatment

1   Adrenaline: 1:1000 solution 0.5-0.7 ml S.C.
2   Promethazine HCl, 50 mg i.v. or chlorpheniramine maleate 10 mg i.v.
3   Hydrocortisone 100 mg i.v.
Should be given in that order. Each may be repeated in 15 minutes if necessary. In addition, the patient should be laid flat with legs elevated, a clear airway established, if necessary by endotracheal tube, and oxygen given by mask if cyanosis develops. The adrenaline is given to counteract small vessel vasodilatation (and the subsequent fall in blood pressure) and bronchoconstriction. Chlorpheniramine and promethezine are antihistamines. The corticosteroid (hydrocortisone) augments the action of adrenaline and reduces the degree of capillary permeability and attendant loss of circulating volume.

Note: similar principles apply to the rare case of anaphylaxis in a dental chair due to insect stings.

5.3   ACUTE RESPIRATORY OBSTRUCTION

Definition

A sudden incapacity on the part of the lungs to maintain normal gaseous exchange owing to obstruction to the upper airways.

Mechanism

In relation to dental practice the common causes are those which lead to

obstruction of pharynx, larynx or trachea,
· Inhalation of a foreign body, e.g. tooth, denture or swab;
· Oedema due to anaphylaxis;
· Facio-maxillary injuries.

With complete obstruction, consciousness is lost in 2-3 min and cardiac arrest occurs within 5-10 min.

Presentation

The cause is usually evident. Acute upper airways obstruction presents with choking, stridor, aphonia, cyanosis and inspiratory indrawing of the chest wall below the level of obstruction.

Management

Simple measures
A sharp slap across the back may cause a sufficiently steep rise in intrathoracic pressure to dislodge an inhaled foreign body. Failing this, the mouth and throat should be examined with the little finger in the hope of "hooking" an impacted solid body.

Laryngoscopy
Provided the instruments can be handled with some skill, the combination of laryngoscope and forceps will retrieve most objects at or above the level of the larynx.

Tracheostomy
Emergency tracheostomy should only be performed where obstruction is complete, simpler measures have failed and the patient is moribund.

Technique: The skin is incised below the larynx and, after palpation, the trachea is opened at least two (cartilage) rings below the cricoid. An alternative is to thrust a needle-mounted canula (e.g. large Medicut) into the trachea at the same level. Although the airflow thus provided will be small, it is usually sufficient to permit a more elective procedure by an experienced surgeon.

Intubation
The use of an endotracheal tube, introduced by laryngoscopy, is more appropriate to some cases of facio-maxillary injury with which the dentist sometimes has to deal. Correct placement of the tube in the trachea (rather than oesophagus) should not be in doubt if introduced under direct vision but can be checked by attempting to inflate the lungs and watching for movement of the chest wall. A common mistake is to use too long a

tube which may pass directly into a main bronchus (usually the right) thus obstructing the other bronchus. A cuffed tube, appropriately inflated after insertion, should be used to prevent subsequent inhalation of blood, debris or vomiting.

Note

The specific management of laryngeal oedema due to anaphylaxis was discussed on p.195. In addition to appropriate drug therapy, intubation and rarely tracheostomy may be required.

5.4   ACUTE ASTHMA

Definition

Acute reversible bronchospasm leading to hypoxia.

Mechanism

Asthma has several causes which may be intrinsic or extrinsic. The final common pathway is probably the release of histamine and other smooth-muscle stimulants (p.84). from local tissue bound mast cells.

Presentation

In the dental chair an asthmatic attack most commonly arises from fear and apprehension although drug reactions (due in particular to penicillin or local anaesthetic injections) may be the precipitant. The patient becomes restless and anxious as the wheeze develops; a few become hysterical. Calm reassurance will sometimes abort the attack. Progressive wheezing may lead to severe air-hunger and cyanosis, which require immediate treatment. Fatalities are rare but are not necessarily related to the duration of the attack; about 15 % of acute asthmatic deaths occur within the first hour of onset.

A panic attack may be distinguished by the lack of wheeze and cyanosis and the presence of gross hyperventilation and physical activity; a bizarre stridor is often present and commonly early signs of tetany (through respiratory alkalosis) develop with paraesthesia in the fingertips and main d'accoucheur.

Note: Early cardiac failure (cardiac asthma) may sometimes be mistaken for true bronchial asthma.

Prevention

A history of asthma should be sought in the clinical assessment. Any drugs known to cause sensitivity reactions should be avoided. Chronic asthma sufferers commonly take regularly prescribed medications and these should not be omitted on the day of dental surgery. Severe asthmatic sufferers taking cortisteroid preparations should increase the oral dose on the day of surgery (p.160) remembering that emotional as well as physical stress may be the cause of a steroid crisis. An intravenous injection of hydrocortisone 100 mg should be given to such patients prior to anything more than the simplest dental procedure.

Management

Calm reassurance is essential. The patient should be allowed to sit upright or slightly forwards to facilitate chest expansion. The following drugs should be used in the acute attack:

Adrenaline
1:1000 solution 0.5-1.0 ml intramuscularly (0.2 ml for small children).

Aminophylline
Failing the desired response to adrenaline, aminophylline (p.86) should be used. A *slow* intravenous injection of 500 mg (250 mg for children) is given.

Hydrocortisone
Should the bronchospasm fail to respond or worsen despite the above measures, particularly in patients with chronic chest disease (e.g. bronchitis or emphysema), hydrocortisone 100 mg i.v. should be given followed by a dextrose or saline infusion providing 100 mg hydrocortisone per hour. (In such an event, of course, medical help should be enlisted immediately.)

Oxygen
Oxygen should be supplied by face mask. 32 % oxygen can be safely given in the initial stages of an acute attack.

5.5   CARDIAC ARREST

Definition

A failure of the heart to pump, due either to cardiac standstill or more commonly to ventricular fibrillation.

Mechanism

Cardiac arrest occurs most commonly as a sequel to myocardial infarction. Most other cases are due to hypoxia, e.g. anaesthetic accidents.

Presentation

Although silent infarctions undoubtedly occur, most are associated with classical anterior chest pain which often radiates into the jaws and upper limbs (commonly the left). Accompanying the infarction pain and breathlessness, sweating and pallor. Cardiac arrest itself is followed immediately by syncope. Commonly there is a deep indrawing of the breath and rolling up of the eyes. The pulse and heart sounds are absent. Respirations may continue for some time.

Management

Irreversible brain damage occurs within three to five minutes unless an adequate circulation is restored. Speed is of the essence. The fact that most cases are the result of ventricular fibrillation rather than irretrievable cardiac damage dictates that resuscitation should always be attempted.

1   Lay the patient flat on the floor with legs elevated to encourage venous return.

2   Clear an airway and remove dentures and other impedimenta. Extend and rotate the neck sideways to prevent inhalation of vomitus. Apply oxygen by mask (p.88).

3   Have an assistant call an ambulance *and* doctor, telling both that cardiac arrest is suspected.

4   Deliver a sharp blow to the praecordium with the fist. This occasionally restores a co-ordinated heart rhythm. Without the luxury of electrocardiographic monitoring and facilities for electrical defibrillation, it is not possible to distinguish fibrillation from cardiac standstill nor effectively to influence the former. The dentist must be content with providing cardiorespiratory support until medical help arrives.

Technique

Place the flat of the right hand over the lower half of the sternum and, kneeling at the side of the patient, deliver five forceful compressions to the chest by placing the heel of the left hand over the knuckles of the right. One's whole body weight should be used. After the fifth compression (about one per second), move to the head of the patient. Close the patient's nostrils with thumb and finger of one hand, at the same time extend the neck and open the mouth by traction of the jaw with the other hand. Inhale deeply and, forming an airtight seal, exhale completely into the patient's lungs. Return to the chest and repeat the cycle. This operation is performed far more efficiently by employing two people and by using an Ambu bag (attached if possible to an oxygen line). This will improve the efficiency of ventilation. Ideally, an endotracheal tube should be inserted but this requires skill and should never compromise the priorities outlined above. If an adequate circulation is restored the patient should not be moved until medical help arrives.

5.6   EPILEPTIC SEIZURE

Definition

Generalised convulsive movements with loss of consciousness (p.186). Seizures, particularly if continuous (status epilepticus) are life-threatening and must be terminated as early as possible.

Mechanism

Epilepsy is only symptomatic if the impulses from a seizure focus are permitted to spread. In dental practice, attacks most frequently result from omission of anticonvulsant drugs the day of dental surgery. The risk is greatest in previously poorly stabilised epileptics and in children. Apprehension, anoxia and pain may all precipitate an attack.

Presentation

Classically the attack starts without warning. The patient may draw a deep breath and become stiff and temporarily apnoeic, often becoming cyanosed (the tonic phase of epilepsy, but check the pulse to distinguish from a cardiac arrest p.198). Within a minute or two the tonic phase gives rise to tremor (clonic phase) frequently generalised but sometimes lateralised or confined to a limb. The patient may pass water and lacerate his tongue. The attack usually terminates spontaneously and a state of post-ictal stupor may develop, sometimes lasting hours.

Prevention

It is clearly vital to elicit a history of epilepsy. Ensure that anticonvulsant drugs are taken early on the day of dental surgery, particularly if general anaesthesia is anticipated as the patient may normally be advised to take nothing, by mouth. If epileptic control has been poor, consult the patient's doctor.

Treatment

1 Remove any impedimenta in the mouth (including dentures).
2 Insert a mouth gag between the teeth.
3 Restrain the patient as necessary and remove any nearby encumbrances on which he may traumatise himself.
4 Inject diazepam 10 mg i.v. if the attack is sustained or recurs.

5.7 TETANY

Definition

Sustained spasm of muscle.

Mechanism

Inadequate plasma level of ionised calcium. Results most frequently from hyperventilation due to apprehension; the loss of CO_2 raises the plasma pH which reduces the level of ionised (though not total) calcium leading to sustained muscle contraction.

Presentation

Hyperventilation is universally present. The patient is usually tense and female. She may complain of dizziness and paraesthesia in the fingers, toes and around the mouth. The slow flexor spasms in the hands (main d'accoucheur) are characteristic and cause considerable distress; hysteria sometimes ensues.

Prevention

Calm reassurance of the tense patient is usually enough.

Treatment

Have the patient breath into a paper or polythene bag, explaining to her the need in order to prevent further apprehension. The procedure increases the level of CO_2 in inspired air and is usually adequate to relieve an attack.

5.8   CONTROL OF DENTAL HAEMORRHAGE
(See also p.171).

Presentation

Usually the result of traumatic extraction, presenting many hours afterwards.

Management

Check medical history for any blood disorder
Remove old blood clot.
Infiltrate local anaesthetic (principally for its vasoconstrictor properties).
Remove any bony spicules
Suture across the socket
Insert an absorbable haemostatic dressing (retained by the suture)
The patient should rest. Mouth rinsing should be avoided
Haemostatic drugs supplement physical means of controlling haemorrhage.

Table 5.1 Haemostatics used in Dental Haemorrhage

Group	Examples	Comment
Vasoconstrictor	Adrenaline in local anaesthetic Adrenaline 1 : 1000 solution applied topically	Vasoconstriction may be followed by reactionary vasodilatation
Absorbable Haemostatic Dressing.	Oxidised regenerated cellulose Gelatin sponge Human fibrin foam	Form a framework for the clot
Thromboplastic Agents	Thrombin Russell's Viper Venom	Easily washed away Liquid applied topically. e.g. on gelatin sponge.
Chemical Styptics	Tannic Acid Ferric Chloride Zinc Chloride	Cause tissue damage Used in gingival retraction cord.
Bone wax	Purified beeswax with additives	Used in periapical surgery. May stimulate a foreign body reaction.

5.9   DRUGS ASSOCIATED WITH EMERGENCIES IN THE DENTAL SURGERY

Extra caution should be taken with patients undergoing medical treatment with the following drugs:

Corticosteroids (p.156)
The stress of major dental surgery may require a temporary increase in dose.

Anticoagulants (p.171).
Dental extractions may lead to protracted bleeding unless prior arrangements are made with the patient's doctor to withdraw one or two doses of the drug.

Oral hypoglycaemic drugs (p.139).
Failure to take usual food on the morning of dental surgery may occasionally lead to hypoglycaemia in patients taking a long half-life drug such as chlorpropamide.

Insulin (p.136).
Liaison must be sought with the patient's doctor. Each diabetic should be considered as an individual and unique case as no two diabetics react in the same way. A dextrose infusion should be available in case of hypoglycaemia.

Hypnotics and sedatives (p.167).
Their effect will add to that of intravenous and inhalation anaesthesia.

PART 6 · SPECIAL TOPICS

6.1   FLUORIDES AND FLUORIDATION

It has long been established that flouride in natural drinking water has an important role to play in the prevention of dental caries; this brief chapter does not aim to detail the immense controversy (much of it emotional rather than scientific) which has hung over the artificial fluoridation of water supplies for so many years; only basic considerations regarding the effects of fluoride on the teeth are considered.

SOURCE OF FLUORIDES

Natural fluorides appear in drinking water as a result of volcanic rock erosion; they are chiefly salts of calcium, iron, aluminium and magnesium. The soil and water content of such flourides varies considerably throughout the world. The first associations between fluoride content of drinking water and dental health were made through epidemiological observation; initially it was noted that areas of abnormally high fluoride content were associated with a high incidence of mottled enamel. At the same time these populations had up to 50 % fewer dental cavities than those from non-fluoride areas. It was established empirically that the optimum concentration of fluoride (i.e. a water content which produced no mottling but prevented caries) was in the region of 1 part per million (1 ppm). A strong case for manipulating the fluoride content of water supplies subsequently developed.

ARTIFICIAL FLUORIDATION

'At source' fluoridation of water supplies has been widely accepted throughout the United States; Europe on the other hand has approached the problem rather more conservatively and most countries have either advocated oral administration or topical application of fluoride or like Britain have introduced fluoridation of the water supplies to selected areas on an experimental basis.

PHARMACOKINETICS OF FLUORIDE

Dietary fluoride is probably absorbed in simple solution by the small intestine. Excretion is chiefly through the kidneys but a proportion may be lost in the sweat. The proportion retained is deposited in the skeleton and soft tissues. The body's intake is higher during growth, pregnancy and lactation.

The highest proportion of fluoride in the body is to be found in bones and teeth where it enters into the apatite structure of the bone salt. The fluoride content of saliva does not vary within the normal range of dietary intake although it is higher in fluorosis areas.

Fluoride is conveyed to foetus and infant via placenta and breast milk.

ACTION OF FLUORIDE ON THE TEETH

1   During calcification: fluoride replaces the hydroxyl ion in hydroxy-apatite forming caries-resistant fluorapatite.
2   After eruption: fluoride is taken up by the enamel surface and may remineralise the early carious lesion.
3   Fluoride ions are enzyme inhibitors and prevent conversion of sugar to acid by the bacteria of dental plaque.

THERAPEUTIC ADMINISTRATION OF FLUORIDES

Tablet
2.2 mg Sodium fluoride (giving an intake of 1 mg).
Half a tablet is taken per day up to age 3.
One tablet per day to age 13 (third molar crown calcified).
The tablet may be chewed (giving a topical effect) as well as swallowed.

Topical Application
2 % Sodium fluoride — a stable solution.
8 or 11 % Stannous fluoride — unstable so must be freshly made.
1.23 % Acidulated phosphate fluoride — solution or gel with applicator tray.
The teeth are carefully polished, one quadrant at a time, dried and the solution applied and left in contact for three or four minutes. The procedure should be repeated every year until adolescence. Zeal matters more than formulation.

Rinsing
0.05 % Sodium fluoride.
Daily rinsing for two minutes — a method suitable for school groups. The solutions used for topical application may also be adapted as rinses.

Fluoride Toothpaste
Sodium fluoride.
Sodium Mono fluorophosphate.
Toothpastes have been less successful than other methods in reducing caries probably due to poor toothbrushing technique.
No standard formulary preparation of fluoride is available in either the Dental Practitioners or the British National Formulary.

Fluoride Toxicity

Acute poisoning
Fluorides in high concentration are irritant and inhibit enzyme systems of the body. Large doses are fatal within two to three days, but acute poisoning is fortunately rare. Nausea, vomiting and abdominal pain lead to muscular weakness and ultimately cardio-respiratory failure.

More commonly poisoning is due to cumulative toxicity in high-fluoride areas.

Chronic poisoning (fluorosis)
When the rate of absorption exceeds that of excretion, cumulative storage of fluoride results. Over-ingestion may result from a high soil and water content of fluoride (endemic fluorosis) or from the environment of certain occupations (industrial fluorosis), where the hazard may involve not only the worker but those living in the neighbourhood of the factory as well.

Endemic fluorosis occurs when the fluoride level in drinking water exceeds two parts per million (2 ppm.) The effects are seen primarily in the teeth of children and in the teeth and skeletons of adults. At levels of fluoride between two and eight ppm, tooth mottling is primarily a cosmetic problem and such teeth are commonly free of caries.

X-rays of bones affected by chronic fluorosis show diffuse osteosclerosis due to increased bone density, and calcification of ligaments and tendons.

6.2   DRUG ABUSE

INTRODUCTION

Acute self-poisoning is at worst a desperate attempt at self-destruction; far more commonly it represents a simple avoidance reaction.

Addiction itself is not a disease, but a symptom of personality defect.

Drug abuse has become a major problem in Western societies. It is not possible in the space available to discuss in any detail the psycho-social aspects, but some of the more important points will be considered.

Abuse takes two forms:
· acute overdosage
· chronic dependence

ACUTE OVERDOSAGE

Whether or not the intent is suicidal, the use of drugs as a pathway to oblivion reflects the fashion of the day rather than the despair of the patient. Corrosive liquids, coal gas ovens and river bridges have all had their vogue, but it is their easy availability in the home which probably accounts for the current popularity of drugs.

Indeed the fashions in prescribing by family doctors are reflected in the particular drugs used by their patients for suicidal or 'parasuicidal' attempts. Barbiturates reached a peak incidence as overdose agents in the early 1960s and have since been displaced by the tricyclic group of anti-depressants.

Clearly two possible solutions to what is now a rapidly escalating problem present themselves.

1   To re-establish a degree of self-reliance in a society which nowadays increasingly turns to medicine at the least sign of stress. (Of course, serious and desperate attempts at suicide do occur but the majority of 'overdoses' are intended to be a means of temporary escape from a stressful situation.)

2   To ensure that safer patterns of prescribing are practised. If an overdose of tablets must (in the patient's view) be taken, it is highly desirable that the drug available to him be as non-toxic as possible. There has undoubtedly been a shift in prescribing habits from barbiturate hypnotics to benzodiazepine drugs such as nitrazepam (from which there has been no authenticated report of death following even massive over-dosage), and it is nowadays difficult to justify the use of barbiturates at all as sleeping tablets. The problem regarding antidepressant drugs, however, continues to worsen.

Diagnosis of acute overdosage

Acute poisoning is common and accounts for over 10 % of hospital admissions. On this basis the finding of drowsiness and coma in young or middle-aged adults in the absence of head injury should be regarded as drug-induced unless proved otherwise. The same applies to children who may rather, however, develop signs of restlessness and excitement.

Treatment

The dentist is unlikely to meet acute drug poisoning but in such an event clearly his responsibilty is to call for medical help and meanwhile to maintain basic life functions. The major threats to life in acute over-dosage are hypoventilation, leading to respiratory failure, hypotension and inhalation of vomit. To minimize these risks the patient should be laid flat on one side, his clothing should be loosened at the collar and his neck slightly extended to permit a free airway. Dentures should be removed and if available oxygen administered via a face mask. Mouth to mouth ventil-ation may be necessary. A quick look round for a bottle may provide the best clue to the particular drug used.

Information regarding toxic effects of ingested drugs, antidotes (where appropriate) and appropriate treatment is available by telephone from government-sponsored poisons information centres in Britain's largest cities.

DRUG DEPENDENCE

Chronic drug dependence presents a different and in many ways a more serious problem than acute overdosage. Dependence may take two forms:

Habituation

Where there is a psychological dependence but no physical need for the drug. Examples include alcohol, tobacco, marihuana, LSD and amphet-amines ('purple hearts', pep-pills).

Addiction

Here there is a physical (metabolic) dependence and sudden withdrawal of the drug can result in a crisis of physical illness. The two most important examples are heroin (diamorphine) and cocaine.

The physical and psychological aspects of dependence are often difficult to distinguish. The decisive factor in the development of addiction is related to the ability of some drugs (such as narcotics) to induce tolerance so that ever increasing doses are required to achieve the same effect.

Patterns of drug dependence
These have changed markedly over the past twenty years. Alcohol still remains the most frequently encountered problem. During the 1950s amphetamines were widely used (and until 1956 were available without

prescription). More recently marihuana and lysergic acid diethylamide (LSD, 'acid') have been taken in increasing quantities. There is fair evidence that chronic use of the latter drugs may·lead some individuals on to heroin and cocaine.

All such drugs are used because of their direct effect upon the central nervous system. They influence mood, perception and ideation all of which may affect behaviour in a deleterious way. It is of the utmost importance to realize that the outcome of experimentation with such drugs depends very much upon the user's personality and its interaction with the effects of the particular drug. It is commonly the immature, unstable personality lacking assurance and self-reliance which first turns to drugs. The young are thus at greatest risk, confronted as they are with immense pressures to conform to the ideals of a modern world.

HABITUATING (HABIT-FORMING) DRUGS

ALCOHOL

The WHO defines alcoholics as:
'Excessive drinkers whose dependence upon alcohol has attained such a degree that they show a noticeable mental disturbance or an interference with bodily or mental health, interpersonal relations, smooth economic and social functioning; or the prodromal signs of such development; they therefore require treatment'.

Kessell and Watson (1965) have suggested three stages in the development of alcohol dependence:
1 Excessive drinking, characterized by tolerance, the feeling of a need to drink in order to perform adequately, socially or at work, and increased guilt feelings.
2 'Addiction', characterized by increased frequency of amnesia, social disruption and lowering of self esteem.
3 Chronic alcoholism. Physical and mental disturbance predominate, tolerance increases further, and delirium tremens (the "DTs") may set in.

Most investigators stress the personality element in alcoholism — 'alcoholism comes in people not in bottles; alcohol cannot be considered the cause of alcoholism any more than petrol can be the cause of automobile accidents (Block 1965)'.

Alcoholism commonly runs in families and drinking patterns, if not inherited, can be 'catching'. Lack of emotional nourishment in childhood is one important factor.

The diagnosis or recognition of the alcoholic depends upon a basic understanding of the personality type and his behaviour. The difference between the compulsive and regular drinker is the loss of control exhibited by the former and his concerted attempts to conceal the habit. There is no such thing as the typical alcoholic but a common pattern can be recognized; his inability to accept frustration and failure to complete objectives — constantly on the defensive — feelings of tension, guilt and resentment — sense of being misunderstood and even persecuted. All alcoholics experience isolation and loneliness overwhelmingly and resort to alcoholic 'binges' during times of stress. Alcohol offers a way out.

The most important type to recognize is the psychopathic alcoholic who through a personality defect (inadequacy) seems plausible and charming yet exhibits gross insincerity and unreliability. He pretends to want help but fails to benefit from past experience and is motivated only to personal advantage. He can be the source of immense social misery to family and relations who unwittingly offer their sympathy, but in fact he benefits neither from their help nor from formal treatment.

Withdrawal symptoms of alcohol

At first there is an increase in pulse rate and mild agitation followed by sweating and tremor. Insomnia is characteristic and there may be fits and hallucinations. Delirium tremens ultimately supervenes when the patient becomes extremely agitated and physically hyperactive.

The treatment of alcoholism is a specialist consideration: it aims at total and permanent abstinence, no middle road.

MARIHUANA

Known colloquially as pot, weed or grass, marihuana is obtained from hemp (cannabis) grown principally in India (hashish), North Africa and the middle East. Its use and importation into Britain and the USA are illegal.

Where the action of amphetamines (see below) is stimulating and energising, that of marihuana is said to calm the mental faculties — 'a drug of peace and contemplation'. In heavy doses it may produce disinhibition, a distorted sense of time and space, illusions and hallucination. Marihuana is commonly taken mixed with tobacco in self-rolled cigarettes (reefers).

By far the most contentious aspect of marihuana is its potential for leading its user on from 'soft' drugs to the 'hard' drugs such as cocaine or heroin. As with alcohol, but to a considerably greater extent, the response to marihuana is closely related to the personality of the user. It is precisely this variation in response which has caused the controversy over legislation on import and consumption. Some claim that prolonged use of marihuana is a sign of instability and that eventually the devotee will seek new adventures with stronger drugs. Another faction argues, probably with equal reason, that marihauna consumption can be easily controlled by the user and is entirely non-addictive. The fact is that a single piece of legislation cannot encompass all possibilites and that while the law forbids its import, the consumption in this country is rising steadily, particularly among the younger generation.

AMPHETAMINES

Unlike the other habituating drugs, amphetamines (i.e. benzedrine and dexedrine) are prescribed therapeutically, though less commonly now than twenty years ago when they first became scheduled drugs.

Amphetamines are the familiar 'pep-pills'. They have a stimulating effect on the user and increase his endurance, albeit temporarily. He experiences a sense of well-being and can keep awake for long hours without need for rest or food. Inevitably the effect eventually wears off leaving a sense of emptiness, rejection and paranoia, known colloquially as 'the horrors'. The only immediate means of regaining a sense of well-being and euphoria is to obtain a further supply of drugs and the cycle becomes continuous.

Amphetamines are used mainly by young people of weak or as yet immature personality, and they seem freely available (at a price) in the night-life of all big cities. There has been much concern about the relationship between the use of amphetamines and criminal acts, though a causal link is difficult to establish when the social background may be the same in both cases. Undoubtedly amphetamines can arouse agression.

Sportsmen have also taken amphetamines to improve endurance although in more recent times commonsense and effective drug-screening procedures have prevailed. Occasionally death through physical exhaustion has attended their use during sporting activities.

LYSERGIC ACID DIETHYLAMIDE (LSD-25)

LSD is a potent hallucinogenic drug which reached its zenith of popularity with the 'flower-people' cult of the Western American seaboard in the 1960s, although it had been introduced much earlier. The new cult attracted many mystical ideologies and was particularly popular among intellectuals, university students and the professional classes. The user of LSD has since gradually descended the social ladder.

LSD is derived from diseased rye and its use, trafficking and importation in both Britain and the USA are illegal. The drug acts powerfully upon the modalities of perception and only microgram quantities are required. It lacks the energizing qualities of amphetamines and calming effects of marihuana; instead it can produce a profound extension of awareness and may seriously distort affect and perception to the point of violence, even homicide.

The classically described hallucinations of colour and light ('of indescribable beauty') are by no means constant and are usually short-lived. Rather more common are reports of a lost sense of reality, loneliness and a frightening kaleidoscope of horrific images from which it is impossible to rid the mind. Nor is the imagery then confined to periods of drug-taking. 'Bad trips' may pervade the user's consciousness at intervals long after the habit has ceased.

In Britain the LSD habit has likewise centred upon college life. Like all psychotropic drugs, it provides an escape from the routines and materialism of modern life, a substitute for spiritual well-being and security.

HARD DRUGS – HEROIN AND COCAINE

Hard drugs are addictive, and if a value judgement can be valid, more dangerous.

Heroin

Heroin is a synthetic agent derived in principle from the alkaloids of the opium poppy grown mainly in South East Asia. Opium was known to the most ancient civilizations and its abuse remains a serious problem to-day.

It was introduced to western medicine from the Middle East during the early middle ages and even today nothing has surpassed the medicinal properties of morphine and heroin (diaminomorphine) in their correct therapeutic context (p.145). Pharmacologically heroin is both a more potent and more rapidly acting drug than morphine but is also more toxic. Even in the therapeutic situation, physical dependence on both drugs rapidly develops and up to twenty times the initial dose may be required within a few days to achieve a satisfactory therapeutic response.

Heroin can be taken orally (as an elixir) but addicts commonly inject the solution intravenously ('mainlining') exposing themselves to the risks of septicaemia, infective endocarditis, and even fatal anaphylaxis. Addicts describe even their first contact with heroin as immensely pleasurable and most have already experienced the less intense effects of 'soft' drugs. In time however, pleasure gives way to driving necessity (the hallmark of addiction) and some will even subject themselves voluntarily to the hell of withdrawal symptoms in order to start again and recapture that initial ecstasy.

The general effect of heroin is to depress physiological function; apnoea can result from excessive dosage. Appetite is suppressed and loss of weight follows. Bodily secretions are diminished and the skin is usually excessively dry. Injection sites are usually obvious on inspection – most commonly the inner aspect of the forearm or the leg (long saphenous vein), just below the knee.

Because of the expense and social isolation engendered by addiction, heroin invariably destroys family, marital and other personal relationships. Its apparently high incidence among the lower social classes is not necessarily a feature of that population group but rather a measure of social decline in the addict.

Withdrawal illness

The characteristic signs of withdrawal illness are probably the means by which heroin addiction is most frequently recognized.

On missing his first 'shot' the addict senses mild distress and agitation accounted for mainly by a psychological fear of what is to come. Within 12 hours he becomes restless and anxious, begins to yawn frequently and breaks out into a profuse sweat; his nose and eyes begin to run. Severe twitching, goose flesh and dilatation of the pupils develop by the first day followed by severe cramps, and generalized hypersecretion which leads to vomiting and diarrhoea. Distress is intense; the pulse rate and blood pressure rise and the blood sugar is elevated.

The height of the syndrome is reached at 48-72 hours after which it subsides, although complete recovery may take months.

Cocaine

Cocaine is at least as old in its origins as opium and is obtained from the leaves of the South American coca shrub. It has been used for centuries by the South American Indian to improve physical endurance but like heroin (with which it usually is taken in combination by addicts) it induces tolerance and is strongly addictive.

Cocaine as used today is a purified alkaloid and was introduced to medicine as a surgical anaesthetic. Its addicts may sniff the powder ('snow') or dilute it for injection. Its extra-medicinal use is illegal in Britain and the USA.

Cocaine is a strong stimulant of the central nervous system. Its action is short-lived and produces intense euphoria followed by a wake of anxiety, fear and somtimes paranoid delusion; it is for this reason that it is usually taken with heroin. It is harmful because of its effect on personality and behaviour which may include acts of unreasoned violence. Addiction to cocaine is becoming less common in Britain although its use among South American natives is parallel to the tabacco habit in 'civilized' societies.

MULTIPLE CHOICE QUESTIONS

PRINCIPLES OF CLINICAL PHARMACOLOGY

1   A drug which is known to have a long plasma t½ (half-life):
1 Will be rapidly excreted
2 May well be strongly protein-bound
3 Will require to be administered infrequently, possibly only once per day.
4 Will almost certainly be lipid-soluble
5 Carries an inherent risk of cumulative toxicity

2   Which of the following would you expect from a lipid soluble drug?
1 Likely to appear in the saliva
2 Poor oral absorption
3 Crosses placenta easily
4 Greater likelihood of toxicity in liver disease
5 Reduced excretion in renal failure

3   Which of these factors may influence the toxicity of a drug?
1 Degree of protein-binding
2 Route of administration
3 Total daily dose
4 The individual to whom the drug is given
5 The introduction of a second drug

4   Aspirin, like many drugs, is a weak acid. Is it likely to be:
1 Better absorbed if given with an alkali
2 More rapidly excreted if the plasma is made more alkaline
3 Metabolised by the liver
4 More rapidly excreted if the patient drinks a lot
5 More toxic in patients with renal failure

5   Highly ionized drugs will tend to be:
1 Poorly absorbed orally
2 Present in breast milk
3 Transferred easily across the blood-brain barrier
4 Distributed into the body's fat
5 Poorly filtered by the renal glomeruli

6   In which of the following situations would you expect the half-life of
    a lipid-soluble, highly protein-bound drug to rise?
    1   Addition of phenylbutazone to the drug regime
    2   Administration of an enzyme-inducing drug
    3   Development of progressive liver cirrhosis
    4   Fall in plasma binding proteins
    5   Untreated myxoedema

7   Which of the following factors directly influence the rate at which a
    drug is absorbed?
    1   The circulation at the site of administration
    2   Absorptive surface area
    3   Volume of total body water
    4   Renal glomerular filtration rate
    5   Route of administration

8   Plasma protein or fixed tissue binding of drugs is important because:
    1   It may greatly reduce the anticipated plasma concentration of a drug
    2   Bound drugs cannot be filtered by the renal glomeruli
    3   A small change in binding may mean an enormous percentage change
    in the plasma concentration of free drug
    4   It accounts for the toxic effects of tetracycline on the teeth
    5   It accounts for the short duration of action of thiopentone

9   A knowledge of drug interactions is important to the dentist because:
    1   Drug interactions are avoidable
    2   Side effects may be prevented
    3   The patient may be unaware of the potential interactions of drugs
    prescribed from other sources
    4   Drugs may otherwise fail to exert their full therapeutic effect
    5   A Court of Law may consider it negligent to prescribe in ignorance
    of such interactions

DENTAL PRESCRIBING

1   Which of the following should be allowed to influence you in the drugs
    you prescribe?
    1   Common sense
    2   Manufacturers' advertising literature
    3   The experience of senior colleagues
    4   Dental Practitioners' Formulary
    5   The drugs the patient is already taking

2   Which of the five 'rules of thumb' referred to in the text and designed
     to reduce iatrogenic disease are present in the following list?
     1 Do not prescribe a drug the metabolism and route of excretion of
     which you are uncertain
     2 Use the lowest effective dose
     3 Use only the dose indicated in the *Dental Practitioners' Formulary*
     4 Continually review the clinical indications for the drug rather than
     repeat prescriptions
     5 Use a minimum number of drugs at any one time

3   Which of the following features will help to identify patients less
     liable to comply with the drugs you prescribe for them?
     1 Old age
     2 Pregnancy
     3 Depression
     4 Failing eyesight
     5 Poor attender for dental appointments

4   A drug is prescribed and fails to produce the intended response. Which
     of the following are likely reasons in practice?
     1 Failure of the patient to take the drug
     2 Thyrotoxicosis
     3 Concurrent administration of other drugs
     4 Malabsorption syndrome
     5 Inadequate dosage

5   Which of the following disorders in childhood should the dentist take
     particular note of when prescribing drugs?
     1 Congenital heart disease
     2 Bronchiectasis
     3 Epilepsy
     4 Acute leukaemia
     5 Coeliac disease

6   Which of the following drugs should be avoided during pregnancy?
     1 Tetracycline
     2 Halothane
     3 Penicillin
     4 Metronidazole
     5 Erythromycin estolate

7   Why are elderly people more susceptible to the adverse reactions of
     drugs?
     1 There are increasing numbers of elderly persons in the population
     2 Cardiac output is reduced in the elderly

3 The elderly are physiologically different from the young

4 Confusion over dosage and drug regimes is more frequent in the elderly

5 The elderly are more likely to be prescribed drug combinations

8 **Which of the following circumstances would influence you to prescribe a drug parenterally rather than orally?**

1 Unreliable patient

2 Emergency

3 Known hypersensitivity to drug

4 The patient is already taking several drugs orally

5 The presence of renal disease

9 **Which of the following are enforceable by Act of Parliament?**

1 A dentist's duty to prescribe where necessary from a list of approved drugs

2 The presentation on request of a register of controlled drugs to an authorised inspector

3 The dentist's personal signature on his own non-scheduled drug prescriptions

4 The reporting of an adverse drug effect to the Medicine's Commission

5 The provision of data sheets to dentists by the pharmaceutical industry

10 **The dentist is not permitted by Law to:**

1 Prescribe Schedule II Drugs

2 Prescribe under any circumstances drugs not listed in the Dental Practitioners' Formulary

3 Store Schedule I Drugs

4 Use National Health Service prescription pads for private patients

5 Prescribe by reference to a previous order

ANAESTHESIA

1 **Which of the following favour a high arterial partial pressure of a general anaesthetic gas?**

1 High inspired concentration

2 High alveolar ventilation

3 High plasma solubility of the gas

4 Low cardiac output

5 High venous partial pressure of the gas

2   **The peak concentration of intravenous anaesthetic reaching the brain depends on:**
     1   Rate of metabolism of the drug
     2   Speed of injection
     3   Heart rate
     4   Site of injection
     5   Dilution of the drug in the syringe

3   **Which indicate that light surgical anaesthesia has been reached or passed?**
     1   Reaction to physical stimulus
     2   Eccentric eyeballs
     3   Paralysis of abdominal musculature
     4   Immobility
     5   Dilated pupil reactive to light

4   **Which are important in the preparation of a patient for a short general anaesthetic?**
     1   A note of current drug therapy
     2   Informed consent of the patient
     3   Pre-operative sedation
     4   Injection of atropine
     5   A careful examination of heart and chest

5   **In a continuous flow anaesthetic machine:**
     1   A flow rate which exceeds the patient's minute volume minimises the risk of accumulating CO_2 in the plasma
     2   A flow rate of 5 litres/minute is usually adequate
     3   A reservoir bag is unnecessary
     4   The expiratory valve should be placed as near to the anaesthetic machine as possible
     5   The ratio of nitrous oxide to oxygen should be maintained at approximately 2:1

6   **The *advantages* of a demand flow over the continuous flow type include:**
     1   It maintains greater accuracy of gas concentration
     2   It can provide a very high flow-rate
     3   It does not require a tight fitting mask
     4   It is less complicated
     5   It can be fitted with a calibrated halothane vapouriser

7   **Nitrous oxide**
     1   Is safe in concentrations exceeding 80%
     2   Cannot produce anaesthesia deeper than Stage 2

3 Is useful in dentistry as an analgesic
4 Is stored as a gas under pressure
5 Is generally used in conjunction with oxygen and halothane

8 Halothane
1 Has good analgesic properties
2 Is a cardiac and respiratory depressant
3 Is liable to cause dysrhythmias
4 Is likely to cause jaundice
5 Can rapidly achieve Stage 3 surgical anaesthesia

9 Intravenous anaesthetics
1 Are all essentially similar in practical usage
2 Cause necrosis if given accidentally into extravascular tissues
3 Are the same as intravenous sedatives
4 Are ideal for conservation work in children
5 May cause anaphylaxis

10 Sedation with intravenous diazepam
1 Differs from anaesthesia in aiming to maintain the patient conscious
2 Potentiates the cerebral depressant action of other drugs
3 Is frequently used in conjunction with local anaesthesia
4 Is very predictable in its effects
5 Is suitable for procedures lasting up to one hour

11 Which are true of pentazocine?
1 An overdose may be reversed immediately by naloxone
2 It may cause withdrawal symptoms in a heroin addict
3 Can be given with complete safety to patients under treatment for blood pressure
4 Should not be administered simultaneously with diazepam
5 It is metabolised within minutes of injection

12 The effectiveness of a local anaesthetic increases with
1 Concentration
2 Solubility in fat
3 Relaxation of the patient
4 Latency period
5 Blood flow at the site of injection

13 Do you agree with the following statements?
1 Lignocaine may cause convulsions
2 Procaine is a vasoconstrictor
3 Felypressin is a sympathomimetic amine
4 Maximum safe dose of lignocaine (with vasoconstrictor) is 400 — 500mg

  5 Adrenaline in local anaesthetics is too dilute to cause systemic toxicity

14 When using lignocaine
  1 You should check for hypersensitivity by first giving a small subcutaneous injection
  2 You should switch to intravenous anaesthesia if the patient is known to be procaine-sensitive
  3 You should not inject a solution more than two months old
  4 A vasoconstrictor is unnecessary
  5 You are using dentistry's most widely used local anaesthetic

15 Vasoconstrictors are useful in local anaesthesia because they —
  1 Permit a smaller volume of local anaesthetic to be used
  2 Reduce bleeding after an extraction
  3 Cause local vasoconstriction at the injection site
  4 Prevent rapid dispersal of the local anaesthetic to nerve endings
  5 Prolong the therapeutic half life of local anaesthetic

16 A 2.2 ml cartridge of 2% lignocaine with adrenaline contains
  1 2.2 mg lignocaine
  2 44 mg lignocaine
  3 2g/100 ml solution
  4 2g/litre solution
  5 Approximately 10% of the toxic dose of lignocaine

ANAEMIA

1 Anaemia
  1 May be present without blood loss and despite normal haemopoiesis
  2 Is a definitive diagnosis
  3 Results from a disturbance in the dynamic balance between red-cell production and breakdown
  4 Is usually a marker of systemic disease
  5 Is often associated with the treatment of inflammatory disorders

2 In the treatment of anaemia
  1 The cause is relatively unimportant
  2 Iron should always be tried in the first instance
  3 Injections every 2 months or so for anaemia usually mean the patient is under treatment for pernicious anaemia
  4 Iron and folate should be given routinely in pregnancy
  5 Phenytoin should ideally be withdrawn

3 Pernicious anaemia
1 Is frequently due to malabsorption syndrome
2 Can be satisfactorily treated with folic acid
3 May sometimes be associated with neurological changes
4 Responds only to vitamin B_{12}
5 Is associated with enamel hypoplasia

4 The following deficiencies may be associated with the combination of pallor and lesions of lips, mouth or tongue.
1 Vitamin B_1
2 Vitamin B_{12}
3 Iron
4 Vitamin C
5 Vitamin D

5 Anaemia may occasionally follow medication with certain —
1 Anticoagulants
2 Anticonvulsants
3 Antihypertensives
4 Antihistamines
5 Anti-inflammatory analgesics

6 Acute blood loss may require immediate treatment by —
1 Plasma expanders
2 Cross-matched whole blood
3 Ferrous sulphate
4 Definitive treatment of the cause
5 Vitamin C

ANGINA

1 Angina
1 Signifies an inadequate supply of oxygen to the myocardium
2 Is usually irreversible
3 May be brought on by factors which increase myocardial tension or contractility
4 May be relieved by agents which reduce myocardial tension or contractility
5 Is a definitive diagnosis

2 Which of the following are likely to reduce sympathetic drive to the heart?
1 Calm reassurance of an anxious patient
2 Sublingual trinitrin (glyceryl trinitrate)

3 Propranolol
4 Physical relaxation
5 Diazepam

3   An attack of angina occurs in the dental chair:
1 It should be regarded as a medical emergency
2 It is best treated with sublingual trinitrin
3 It might be avoided on the next occasion by prophylactic use of trinitrin
4 The patient should be sat in an upright position
5 The patient's general practitioner should be contacted routinely

HYPERTENSION

1   An elevation in blood pressure may result from
1 Peripheral vasoconstriction
2 Rise in heart rate
3 Rise in cardiac stroke volume
4 Increased sympathetic drive to the heart
5 The use of sodium-retaining drugs

2   Drugs used to treat hypertension may act in which of the following ways
1 By reducing cardiac stroke volume
2 By reducing heart rate
3 By stimulating renal release of renin
4 By reducing peripheral resistance
5 By reducing autonomic outflow from the CNS

3   The major problems with post-ganglion adrenergic neurone blocking drugs include
1 Postural hypotension on raising the patient from a horizontal dental chair
2 Extreme sensitivity of the patient to the quantities of adrenaline used in local anaesthesia
3 Immune haemolytic anaemia
4 Weakness
5 Depression

4   Which of the following drugs should be used with great caution in patients already taking antihypertensive agents.
1 Proprietary cold cures
2 Imipramine
3 Carbenoxolone
4 Chlorpromazine
5 Halothane

HEART FAILURE

1 Systemic oedema may be associated with
1 Rise in capillary hydrostatic pressure
2 Normal circulating blood volume
3 Reduced circulating blood volume
4 Hyperaldosteronism
5 High plasma renin

2 Treatment for heart failure is aimed at reducing
1 Plasma renin levels
2 Sodium retention
3 Pump failure
4 Sympathetic drive to the heart
5 Aldosterone levels

3 The actions of digoxin which are useful in treating simple heart failure include
1 Decrease in atrial refractory period
2 Improvement in renal plasma flow
3 Increase in myocardial excitability
4 Increase in myocardial contractility
5 Depression of conducting tissue

4 The factors commonly contributing to digoxin toxicity include
1 Old age
2 Poor renal function
3 Interaction with highly protein-bound drugs
4 General anaesthesia
5 Fall in plasma potassium levels

5 Loop diuretics are very powerful because
1 They cause the loss of more water than salt
2 They act on the loop of Henle
3 They destroy the counter-current mechanism
4 They encourage loss of potassium from the body
5 They prevent resorption of water from the distal tubule and collecting ducts

6 Common effects of digoxin toxicity include
1 Dizziness
2 Nausea
3 Irregularity of the pulse
4 Tremor
5 Loss of appetite

7 **Patients on thiazide diuretics may complain of**
1 Muscular weakness
2 Gouty arthritis
3 Dizziness on switching suddenly from the horizontal to the vertical position
4 Increase in dental caries
5 More intense side effects from digoxin

8 **The following are drugs used in the treatment of heart failure**
1 Aminophylline suppositories
2 Chlorothiazide
3 Potassium chloride
4 Terbutaline sulphate
5 Procainamide

9 **Spironolactone**
1 Is a powerful diuretic
2 Requires potassium supplements
3 Antagonises aldosterone action
4 Is usually used to complement other diuretics
5 Should not be given in renal failure

RESPIRATORY DISEASE

1 **The plasma Pco_2 will tend to rise**
1 In pulmonary congestion due to heart failure
2 After a pneumonectomy (removal of one lung)
3 During oversedation with intravenous diazepam
4 With excessive 'dead-space' in an anaesthetic machine
5 In chronic obstructive airways disease

2 **The following drugs may be useful in reversing an acute attack of bronchial asthma**
1 Adrenaline
2 Terbutaline
3 Antihistamines
4 Sodium cromoglycate
5 Beclomethasone

3 **Chronic bronchitis is characterised by**
1 Raised pCo_2
2 Excessive amounts of sputum which can be effectively cleared by mucolytic drugs
3 Recurrent infections which can be effectively treated by antibiotics

4 Bronchoconstriction which can be effectively reversed by β-adrenergic stimulant drugs

5 Chronic hypoxia

4   The chronic bronchitic who develops acute breathlessness following a paroxysm of coughing might be helped with

1 An 'MC' mask switched down to 2 litres/minute of oxygen

2 A '28%' venti-mask

3 Injection of an analeptic

4 Sitting in the upright position

5 A dose of a cough suppressant

5   Ephedrine

1 Acts as a decongestant by causing vasoconstriction when applied to the nasal mucosa

2 Exerts a stimulant effect on the CNS

3 May cause insomnia

4 Is a drug of addiction

5 Antagonises noradrenaline

DYSRHYTHMIAS

1   Dysrhythmias

1 May be caused by the drugs used to treat them

2 May result from too much atropine in a premedicant

3 Are logically treated by drugs which block β-adrenoceptors

4 Are potentiated by halothane

5 Are frequently triggered by the adrenaline vasoconstrictor in a local anaesthetic

2   Adrenergic stimulation of the heart

1 Causes instability of the membrane potential

2 Increases the tendency to automaticity

3 May lead to heart block

4 May be blocked by propranolol

5 May be reduced by calm reassurance

3 β-adrenoceptor blockers are risky in which situation?

1 Chronic bronchitis because bronchial patency depends on sympathetic drive

2 Incipient pulmonary oedema because cardiac performance depends on sympathetic drive

3 A stressful dental appointment because emotional calm depends on autonomic activity

4 Diabetes because the signs of over treatment (hypoglycaemia) depend on sympathetic action

5 General anaesthesia because blood pressure reflexes depend on sympathetic action

4   **A patient develops a rapid tachycardia but remains fully conscious following injection of a local anaesthetic with adrenaline. You should**
     1 Phone for an ambulance immediately
     2 Wait a few minutes in the hope that the heart will revert back to normal rhythm
     3 Inject some plain lignocaine intravenously in the knowledge that it suppresses spontaneous pacemaker activity
     4 Try rubbing the carotid sinus on one side of the neck
     5 Make a point of using an aspirating syringe on the next occasion

ORAL ULCERATION

1   **Oral ulceration**
     1 Is usually traumatic in origin
     2 Should be viewed suspiciously if it fails to resolve in 2-3 weeks
     3 May be an early indication of systemic disease
     4 Usually responds to symptomatic treatment
     5 Should be biopsied routinely

2   **In apthous ulceration**
     1 There are as many treatments as there are theories of aetiology
     2 The lesions heal with or without treatment
     3 Steroids are the drugs of choice
     4 The major symptom requiring treatment is pain
     5 Recurrences may be prevented by appropriate drugs

3   **The following are important in the management of acute ulcerative gingivitis.**
     1 Tincture of silver nitrate, neutralised with eugenol
     2 Penicillin lozenges
     3 Metronidazole
     4 Mouthwashes
     5 Idoxuridine

4   **Specific treatment is available for the following oral conditions.**
     1 Established cold sore
     2 Oral thrush
     3 Lichen planus
     4 Erythema multiforme
     5 Primary chancre

5 **The following conditions may be symptomatic of adverse reaction to systemic drug therapy.**
  1 Dental caries
  2 Gingivitis
  3 Mouth ulcers
  4 Skin rash
  5 Enamel hypoplasia

GASTRO-INTESTINAL DISORDERS

1 **Drugs are used in the treatment of peptic ulcer**
  1 To neutralise gastric acid
  2 To inhibit secretion of stomach acid
  3 To avert a metabolic acidosis
  4 To improve the quality of mucin
  5 To suppress the patient's appetite

2 **The following drugs are curative rather than symptomatic in the treatment of peptic ulcer**
  1 Magnesium trisilicate
  2 Cimetidine
  3 Aluminium hydroxide
  4 Propantheline
  5 Carbenoxolone

3 **Diarrhoea may result from**
  1 Treatment with tetracycline
  2 Codeine phosphate
  3 Chronic use of Epsom Salts
  4 Kaolin and morphine mixture
  5 Drugs used in the treatment of simple anaemia

INFECTION

1 **Chemotherapeutic agents are**
  1 Generally free of side effects
  2 Only effective if bactericidal
  3 Limited in use by the development of bacterial resistance
  4 Generally over prescribed
  5 Relatively ineffective against viruses

2 Lack of response to an antimicrobial may be due to
1 Failure of the patient to follow instructions
2 Infection by a virulent organism
3 Use of an oral preparation
4 Need for surgical intervention
5 Combining bactericidal and bacteristatic drugs

3 The choice of antibiotic should be influenced by
1 Pharmaceutical data sheets
2 Clinical signs of the infection
3 Cost
4 Posititive bacteriological identification
5 The presence of renal disease

4 Penicillin
1 Cannot be synthesised
2 Destroys Gram +ve cocci
3 May cause glossitis
4 Cannot be given in depot form
5 May be the cause of an itchy rash

5 A patient with a systolic heart murmur requires an extraction. The last time an extraction was performed (under penicillin cover) an itchy rash developed.
1 No antibiotic should be given
2 Use tetracycline in place of penicillin
3 Give penicillin and refer the patient to his doctor for the rash
4 Give erythromycin 250mg orally for 5 days before the extraction
5 Give erythromycin 500mg I.M. one hour before extraction and 250mg tablets for 5 days afterwards

6 Tetracyclinc staining of teeth
1 Is easily polished off
2 Can be used to date the administration of tetracycline
3 Is most noticeable if the drug has been given between the ages of 6 months and 6 years
4 Does not affect decidous teeth
5 Varies in colour and intensity according to the type of tetracycline

7 Sulphonamide − containing drugs
1 No longer have a place in modern practice
2 Are used in maxillo-facial surgery
3 Are antagonised by procaine
4 Must be avoided in patients with urinary infections
5 May cause pancytopoenia

8 **Denture sore mouth**
   1 Is a form of oral moniliasis
   2 Follows prolonged antibiotic therapy
   3 Is cured by administering nystatin or amphotericin
   4 Is due to allergy to the denture base material
   5 Is due to oral neglect

9 **Triplopen**
   1 Provides an immediate high plasma level of penicillin
   2 Acts for 2-3 days
   3 Reduces the risk of anaphylaxis
   4 Is useful for unreliable patients
   5 Is suitable for prophylaxis against infective endocarditis

10 **Disinfectant solutions**
   1 Are routinely used to sterilise dental instruments
   2 Cannot penetrate blood and saliva stains
   3 Must be supplemented by soap
   4 Have constantly to be made up and replaced
   5 May support the growth of virulent pathogens

11 **The choice of disinfectant depends on**
   1 The material to be disinfected
   2 The time available
   3 The presence of organic residue
   4 Cost
   5 Expert bacteriological advice

ENDOCRINE DISORDERS

1 **The following endocrine glands are subject to pituitary stimulation.**
   1 Thyroid
   2 Parathyroid
   3 Adrenal
   4 Pancreatic Islet (B cells)
   5 Mammary

2 **Which of the following will reduce the circulating levels of thyroid hormone in thyrotoxicosis?**
   1 Surgery
   2 Radioactive iodine
   3 β-adrenoceptor blockers
   4 Potassium perchlorate
   5 Carbimazole

3   **A patient with Addison's disease**
    1 Requires replacement steroid therapy
    2 May collapse if subjected to a stressful dental procedure
    3 Is prone to spreading infections
    4 Will require a booster dose of steroid for conservation work
    5 Will require a booster dose of steroid for an extraction

4   **Oral contraceptives (containing oestrogen)**
    1 Are widely used
    2 Are a recognised cause of hypertension
    3 Should be stopped one month prior to a dental general anaesthetic
    4 Increase the incidence of venous thrombosis
    5 May cause chronic marginal gingivitis

5   **Insulin**
    1 Requirements are proportional to carbohydrate intake
    2 Permits uptake of glucose by muscle, fat and liver cells
    3 Is destroyed by gastric enzymes
    4 Is potentiated by adrenaline
    5 Can be antigenic

6   **A diabetic taking insulin zinc suspension (Lente) requires a general anaesthetic for the extraction of an abscessed tooth. You should**
    1 Increase his insulin dose on the day of operation
    2 Admit patient to hospital and change to soluble insulin
    3 Take insulin as usual but delay breakfast till after the anaesthetic
    4 Delay both insulin and breakfast till after the procedure
    5 Monitor the blood sugar

7   **The following are complications of replacement therapy with adrenal corticosteroids**
    1 Excessive weight gain
    2 Hypertension
    3 Abdominal striae
    4 Excessive sweating
    5 Irritability

PAIN

1   **In the effective management of pain**
    1 The cause is relatively unimportant
    2 Anti-inflammatory drugs tend to offer higher analgesic potency than simple pain killers
    3 Psychology is important

    4 Chlorpromazine may be a useful adjunct to analgesic drugs
    5 Pentazocine should be given initially

2 Codeine
    1 Is related to the narcotic analgesics
    2 Is liable to cause diarrhoea
    3 Is a potent analgesic
    4 Is a useful cough suppressant
    5 Is frequently mixed with aspirin in proprietary pain-killers

3 Which of the following might lead you to prescribe paracetamol rather than aspirin for a patient with mild toothache.
    1 Recent myocardial infarction
    2 Taking warfarin after sustaining a deep vein thrombosis
    3 An overdose of aspirin 6 months ago
    4 Recently diagnosed duodenal ulcer
    5 Known case of gouty arthritis

4 Which of the following are salient differences between narcotic and non-narcotic analgesics?
    1 Tolerance
    2 Cerebral depressant action
    3 Power of analgesia
    4 Action reversible by naloxone
    5 Can induce sleep

5 Pethidine
    1 Can be prescribed by a dentist on an NHS prescription
    2 Is a powerful constipant
    3 Has a useful euphoriant effect
    4 Is addictive over a period of time
    5 May cause respiratory depression

6 Paracetamol is widely used as a routine analgesic because it
    1 Is virtually non-toxic whatever the dose
    2 Has no anti-inflammatory action
    3 It does not cause gastro-intestinal upset
    4 Has a stronger analgesic action than aspirin
    5 Requires only to be taken twice daily

INFLAMMATION

1 As a group, anti-inflammatory drugs
    1 Are generally less toxic than simple pain-killers

  2 Tend to influence only pathological (as opposed to protective) inflammation
  3 Are seldom able to relieve pain effectively
  4 Have very considerable therapeutic value
  5 Are all basically anti-histamines

2   The primary actions of salicylates are
  1 Antipyretic
  2 Anti-inflammatory
  3 Gastric irritant
  4 Hypersensitivity
  5 Analgesic

3   Which of the following anti-inflammatory drugs should be avoided in patients taking warfarin (oral anti-coagulant)?
  1 Aspirin
  2 Phenylbutazone
  3 Mefenamic acid
  4 Naproxen
  5 Indomethacin

4   Phenylbutazone
  1 Is a weak analgesic
  2 May be effective in tempero-mandibular arthritis
  3 Is a potent enzyme inducer
  4 Is currently the commonest cause of drug-induced aplastic anaemia
  5 Is not liable to cause gastric haemorrhage

5   Topical steroids used for oral lesions
  1 Are unlikely to be significantly absorbed
  2 Are hazardous and should not be prescribed
  3 Are usually prescribed to relieve pain
  4 Should be increased at times of stress
  5 Reduce the healing time dramatically

6   Which of the following are toxic effects of long-term pharmacological doses of corticosteroids.
  1 Retardation of growth in children
  2 Tendency to attacks of hypoglycaemia
  3 Formation of cataracts
  4 Dry socket
  5 Osteoporosis

7 Prior to dental extraction under anaesthesia, which of the following preparations should be made for the patient on chronic treatment with systemic corticosteroids.
1 The patient should always be referred to a dental hospital or hospital dental clinic
2 Injectable hydrocortisone ampoules should be readily available
3 100 − 200mg hydrocortisone IV should be given immediately before the procedure
4 A continuous infusion of hydrocortisone should be made up if surgery becomes prolonged
5 Precautions should be taken even six months after withdrawal of long term steroids

8 Antihistamines
1 Are dangerous for the patient who drives a vehicle
2 Are useful in the treatment of peptic ulcer due to excessive gastric acid
3 Are only of therapeutic use as anti-inflammatory agents in anaphylaxis
4 Are potent enzyme-inducers
5 May cause dry mouth

DEPRESSION

1 As a dentist
1 You are unlikely to meet patients on drug treatment for depression unless you work in a psychiatric institution
2 The side effects of antidepressant drugs are of little relevance to your work
3 You should avoid general anaesthesia in patients on anti-depressant drugs
4 You should be aware that self-neglect is frequently a symptom of depression
5 You should consider whether the depressed patient is less likely to comply with the drugs you prescribe

2 Which of the following is true of the endogenously depressed patient on a tricyclic antidepressant?
1 He may present to the dentist complaining of an intolerably dry mouth
2 He should avoid local anaesthetics containing adrenaline
3 He may react unfavourably to certain anti-hypertensive drugs
4 He should avoid meat extracts
5 He has an 80% chance of relief from his symptoms

3   Tricyclic antidepressants may interact unfavourably with the following drugs
1 Mono-amine oxidase inhibitors
2 Pethidine
3 Cephalosporins
4 Benzodiazepines
5 General anaesthetics

4   Signs of excessive dose of tricyclic antidepressants include
1 Bradycardia
2 Elation
3 Mydriasis
4 Excessive sweating
5 Tremor

INSOMNIA and ANXIETY

1   Hypnotic drugs
1 Are frequently habituating
2 Induce natural sleep
3 Frequently differ from tranquillizers only in the dose administered
4 Potentiate intravenous sedation (anaesthesia)
5 Can be withdrawn suddenly without harm to the patient

2   Which of the following are true for the patient taking a phenothiazine drug
1 He is likely to be suffering from a psychotic illness
2 He is liable to be very sensitive to general anaesthetics
3 He has a greater than random chance of developing jaundice
4 He may faint on rising suddenly from a horizontal position
5 He may develop facial 'tics' and spasms as a side-effect of the drug

3   Barbiturates
1 Should be reserved exclusively for the treatment of epilepsy
2 Frequently reduce the plasma levels of other protein-bound drugs
3 Are superior to benzodiazepines as hypnotics
4 Exhibit tolerance
5 Are addictive

4   Benzodiazepines (e.g. diazepam, nitrazepam)
1 Are placed in the group of major 'tranquillizers'
2 Are anticonvulsive
3 Have a very high margin of safety (therapeutic ratio)
4 Cause forgetfulness if taken long-term
5 Can be a threat to safe driving

THROMBO-EMBOLISM and
HEREDITARY HAEMORRHAGIC DISORDERS

1   **Which may predispose to thrombosis?**
    1 Tissue damage
    2 Deficiency of vitamin K
    3 Oestrogen-containing contraceptive pills
    4 Blood stasis
    5 An excess of plasminogen activator

2   **Which of the following drugs may interact with Warfarin?**
    1 Phenylbutazone
    2 Aspirin
    3 Benzylpenicillin
    4 Barbiturate sedatives
    5 Indomethacin

3   **Which reduce the tendency to bleed?**
    1 Antihaemophilic globulin
    2 Epsilon-amino-caproic acid
    3 Streptokinase
    4 Vitamin K
    5 Phenindione

4   **Which are appropriate to management of haemophilia?**
    1 Transfusion of stored blood
    2 Epsilon-amino-caproic acid
    3 Thrombin packs
    4 Factor IX
    5 Plasma cryoprecipitate

5   **Which factors may help in distinguishing haemophilia from von Willebrand's disease?**
    1 Excessive bleeding with even mild trauma
    2 Deficiency of factor VIII
    3 Sex of the patient
    4 Response to corticosteroids
    5 Bleeding tendency in the mother

6   **An emergency extraction is required for a patient taking Warfarin as a prophylactic against myocardial infarction**
    1 Contact the patient's physician
    2 Refer the patient to a hospital
    3 Stop the anticoagulant prior to extraction
    4 Give vitamin K prior to the extraction
    5 Extract the tooth and suture the socket

MALIGANT DISEASE

1   Which of the following are currently the three main approaches to the treatment of malignancy
1 Radiation
2 Immunotherapy
3 Surgical resection
4 Cytotoxic drugs
5 Corticosteroid drugs

2   Which of the following malignancies may currently be considered curable in a majority of cases
1 Acute lymphoblastic leukaemia
2 Chronic lymphatic leukaemia
3 Carcinoma prostate
4 Early Hodgkin's disease
5 Carcinoma lung

3   Which are virtually inevitable side effects of cytotoxic drugs?
1 Candida infection of the mouth (thrush)
2 Anaemia
3 Progressive periodontal disease
4 Faucial ulceration
5 Undue haemorrhage after extractions

4   What should be uppermost in the dentist's mind when asked to consider extractions in a patient undergoing treatment for multiple myeloma
1 Life expectancy of the patient
2 The problems of potential haemorrhage
3 The risk to the patient of dental sepsis if the teeth remain
4 The possibility of pathological fractures of the mandible resulting from myelomatous lesions
5 The haemoglobin level

5   Which are established principles of drug treatment of leukaemias and lymphomas?
1 The therapeutic ratio of drugs in combination is higher than that of drugs used alone
2 Cellular resistance to drugs can be reduced by drug rotation
3 The intermittent use of drugs may be more effective than daily administration
4 Blood transfusions are avoided owing to the risk of infection
5 Corticosteroids are used primarily for their cytoreductive effect on lymphocytes

EPILEPSY

1 **Phenytoin**
  1 Is the most widely effective anticonvulsant drug
  2 May cause severe gingival hyperplasia in the edentulous
  3 Is particularly useful because it lacks sedative action
  4 May cause staggering
  5 Can safely be omitted the day of dental surgery in epileptic children

2 **Epilepsy**
  1 Is always associated with convulsive movements
  2 Is treated optimally in the long term by trial and error with different anticonvulsant drugs
  3 May not involve loss of consciousness
  4 Is best treated by intravenous diazepam when multiple convulsions occur
  5 Can be precipitated by the dentist

3 **Which of the following are recognised precipitants of grand mal attack?**
  1 Fever
  2 Alcohol
  3 Watching TV
  4 Insulin 'reaction'
  5 Apprehension

VITAMIN DEFICIENCY STATE

1 **Which of the following statements do you believe to be true regarding vitamins**
  1 Vitamins are vital to normal metabolism
  2 Clinical deficiency is common in the U.K.
  3 Vitamin tablets should be taken daily for optimum health
  4 An excess of vitamins is harmless
  5 They have an immense placebo value

2 **Specific vitamins are commonly of therapeutic or prophylactic value in which of the following situations?**
  1 Osteomalacia (rickets in children)
  2 Hypoparathyroidism
  3 Fatigue
  4 Infants on powdered milk
  5 Dental hypocalcification

3 Which of the following contribute to the toxicity of excess vitamin D?
1 It is cumulative
2 It mobilises calcium from bones
3 It is metabolised by the kidney
4 Its action may be delayed several months
5 It increases gastro-intestinal absorption of calcium

MEDICAL EMERGENCIES

1 When faced with a serious medical emergency in your surgery, would you say that
1 A successful outcome is more likely to result from application of common sense rather than a detailed medical knowledge
2 Your duty is to act positively rather than retreat from the situation, even though you may be unsure of the diagnosis
3 Failure to have a stock of emergency drugs available is tantamount to negligence
4 Hysteria is the most likely underlying cause
5 It might well have been preventable had a more complete medical and drug history been taken

2 Which of the following drugs can cause a medical emergency in the dental surgery?
1 Prednisolone
2 Phenytoin
3 Chlorpropamide
4 Quinalbarbitone
5 Warfarin

3 A patient to whom you are about to administer a local anaesthetic becomes restless and wheezy: would this likely be due to
1 A heart attack (coronary thrombosis)
2 An anaphylactic reaction to the anaesthetic
3 Hypoglycaemia
4 Asthma
5 Panic attack

4 In a case of suspected 'cardiac arrest'
1 Anginal pain usually precedes the arrest
2 Heart sounds and pulse are absent
3 A doctor should be called right away
4 Irreversible brain damage occurs within 1 minute of 'arrest'
5 The myocardium is often irretrievably damaged if the suspicion is correct

5   The following drugs are frequently the cause of systemic anaphylaxis
     1 Triamcinolone
     2 Aspirin
     3 Diazepam
     4 Procaine
     5 Penicillin

FLUORIDES and FLUORIDATION

1   **Fluoride salts**
     1 Do not occur naturally in drinking water
     2 Are never toxic unless administered through artificial fluoridation
     programmes
     3 Can disfigure tooth enamel
     4 Exert an optimum effect on the teeth at a concentration of 1 ppm
     5 Are harmless at a concentration of 1 ppm

2   **Fluoride salts may be administered**
     1 By mouth rinses of sodium fluoride
     2 By incorporation into toothpastes
     3 By painting directly on to teeth
     4 By swallowing tablets
     5 By depot injection

3   **When advising your patient about the use of fluorides, would you say
     that**
     1 Oral hygiene is more important than fluoridation of public water
     supplies
     2 Persistence with a fluoride preparation is more important than its
     formulation
     3 Excessive ingestion of fluoride salts by a pregnant mother may
     disfigure the infant's primary teeth
     4 The arguments against fluoridation of water supplies are ethical
     rather than scientific
     5 Fluoride protects only children's teeth

ANSWERS TO
MULTIPLE CHOICE QUESTIONS

PRINCIPLES OF CLINICAL PHARMACOLOGY

1	1 No	2 Yes	3 Yes	4 No	5 Yes
2	1 Yes	2 No	3 Yes	4 Yes	5 No
3	1 Yes	2 Yes	3 Yes	4 Yes	5 Yes
4	1 No	2 Yes	3 No	4 Yes	5 Yes
5	1 Yes	2 No	3 No	4 No	5 No
6	1 No	2 No	3 Yes	4 No	5 Yes
7	1 Yes	2 Yes	3 No	4 No	5 Yes
8	1 Yes	2 Yes	3 Yes	4 Yes	5 Yes
9	1 Yes	2 Yes	3 Yes	4 Yes	5 Yes

DENTAL PRESCRIBING

1	1 Yes	2 No	3 Yes	4 Yes	5 Yes
2	1 Yes	2 Yes	3 No	4 Yes	5 Yes
3	1 Yes	2 No	3 Yes	4 Yes	5 Yes
4	1 Yes	2 No	3 Yes	4 No	5 Yes
5	1 Yes	2 No	3 Yes	4 Yes	5 No
6	1 Yes	2 No	3 No	4 No	5 Yes
7	1 No	2 No	3 Yes	4 Yes	5 Yes
8	1 Yes	2 Yes	3 No	4 No	5 No
9	1 Yes	2 Yes	3 No	4 No	5 Yes
10	1 No	2 No	3 No	4 Yes	5 Yes

ANAESTHESIA

1	1 Yes	2 Yes	3 No	4 Yes	5 No
2	1 No	2 Yes	3 Yes	4 Yes	5 Yes
3	1 No	2 No	3 Yes	4 Yes	5 No
4	1 Yes	2 Yes	3 No	4 No	5 Yes
5	1 Yes	2 No	3 No	4 No	5 Yes
6	1 No	2 Yes	3 No	4 No	5 No
7	1 No	2 Yes	3 Yes	4 No	5 Yes
8	1 No	2 Yes	3 Yes	4 No	5 Yes
9	1 Yes	2 No	3 No	4 No	5 Yes
10	1 Yes	2 Yes	3 Yes	4 No	5 Yes

11	1 Yes	2 Yes	3 No	4 No	5 No
12	1 Yes	2 Yes	3 Yes	4 No	5 No
13	1 Yes	2 No	3 No	4 Yes	5 No
14	1 No	2 No	3 No	4 No	5 Yes
15	1 Yes	2 Yes	3 Yes	4 No	5 Yes
16	1 No	2 Yes	3 Yes	4 No	5 Yes

ANAEMIA

1	1 Yes	2 No	3 Yes	4 No	5 Yes
2	1 No	2 No	3 Yes	4 Yes	5 No
3	1 No	2 No	3 Yes	4 No	5 No
4	1 No	2 Yes	3 Yes	4 Yes	5 No
5	1 Yes	2 Yes	3 Yes	4 No	5 Yes
6	1 Yes	2 Yes	3 No	4 Yes	5 No

ANGINA

1	1 Yes	2 No	3 Yes	4 Yes	5 No
2	1 Yes	2 No	3 Yes	4 Yes	5 Yes
3	1 Yes	2 Yes	3 Yes	4 Yes	5 No

HYPERTENSION

1	1 Yes	2 Yes	3 Yes	4 Yes	5 Yes
2	1 Yes	2 Yes	3 No	4 Yes	5 Yes
3	1 Yes	2 No	3 No	4 Yes	5 Yes
4	1 Yes	2 Yes	3 No	4 Yes	5 Yes

HEART FAILURE

1	1 Yes	2 No	3 No	4 Yes	5 Yes
2	1 No	2 Yes	3 Yes	4 No	5 No
3	1 No	2 Yes	3 No	4 Yes	5 No
4	1 Yes	2 Yes	3 No	4 No	5 Yes
5	1 No	2 Yes	3 Yes	4 No	5 Yes
6	1 No	2 Yes	3 Yes	4 No	5 Yes
7	1 Yes	2 Yes	3 Yes	4 No	5 Yes
8	1 Yes	2 Yes	3 Yes	4 No	5 No
9	1 No	2 No	3 Yes	4 Yes	5 Yes

RESPIRATORY DISEASE

	1		2		3		4		5	
1	1	No	2	No	3	Yes	4	Yes	5	Yes
2	1	Yes	2	Yes	3	No	4	No	5	No
3	1	No	2	No	3	Yes	4	No	5	Yes
4	1	No	2	Yes	3	No	4	Yes	5	No
5	1	Yes	2	Yes	3	Yes	4	No	5	No

DYSRHYTHMIAS

	1		2		3		4		5	
1	1	Yes	2	Yes	3	Yes	4	Yes	5	No
2	1	Yes	2	Yes	3	No	4	Yes	5	Yes
3	1	Yes	2	Yes	3	No	4	Yes	5	Yes
4	1	No	2	Yes	3	No	4	Yes	5	Yes

ORAL ULCERATION

	1		2		3		4		5	
1	1	Yes	2	Yes	3	Yes	4	Yes	5	No
2	1	Yes	2	Yes	3	No	4	Yes	5	No
3	1	No	2	No	3	Yes	4	Yes	5	No
4	1	No	2	Yes	3	No	4	No	5	Yes
5	1	Yes	2	Yes	3	Yes	4	Yes	5	Yes

GASTRO-INTESTINAL DISORDERS

	1		2		3		4		5	
1	1	Yes	2	Yes	3	No	4	Yes	5	No
2	1	No	2	Yes	3	No	4	No	5	Yes
3	1	Yes	2	No	3	Yes	4	No	5	Yes

INFECTION

	1		2		3		4		5	
1	1	No	2	No	3	Yes	4	Yes	5	Yes
2	1	Yes	2	Yes	3	No	4	Yes	5	Yes
3	1	Yes	2	Yes	3	Yes	4	Yes	5	Yes
4	1	No	2	Yes	3	Yes	4	No	5	Yes
5	1	No	2	No	3	No	4	No	5	Yes
6	1	No	2	Yes	3	Yes	4	No	5	Yes
7	1	No	2	Yes	3	Yes	4	No	5	Yes
8	1	Yes	2	Yes	3	No	4	No	5	Yes
9	1	No	2	Yes	3	No	4	Yes	5	No
10	1	No	2	Yes	3	No	4	Yes	5	Yes
11	1	Yes	2	Yes	3	Yes	4	Yes	5	Yes

ENDOCRINE DISORDERS

	1		2		3		4		5
1	1 Yes	2 No	3 Yes	4 No	5 Yes
2	1 Yes	2 Yes	3 No	4 Yes	5 Yes
3	1 Yes	2 Yes	3 No	4 No	5 Yes
4	1 Yes	2 Yes	3 No	4 Yes	5 Yes
5	1 Yes	2 Yes	3 Yes	4 No	5 Yes
6	1 No	2 No	3 No	4 Yes	5 No
7	1 No	2 No	3 No	4 No	5 No

PAIN

1	1 No	2 No	3 Yes	4 Yes	5 No
2	1 No	2 No	3 No	4 Yes	5 Yes
3	1 No	2 Yes	3 No	4 Yes	5 Yes
4	1 Yes	2 Yes	3 No	4 No	5 No
5	1 No	2 No	3 Yes	4 Yes	5 Yes
6	1 No	2 Yes	3 Yes	4 No	5 No

INFLAMMATION

1	1 No	2 No	3 No	4 Yes	5 No
2	1 Yes	2 Yes	3 No	4 No	5 Yes
3	1 Yes	2 Yes	3 Yes	4 Yes	5 Yes
4	1 Yes	2 Yes	3 Yes	4 Yes	5 No
5	1 Yes	2 No	3 Yes	4 No	5 No
6	1 Yes	2 No	3 No	4 No	5 Yes
7	1 No	2 Yes	3 Yes	4 Yes	5 Yes
8	1 Yes	2 No	3 Yes	4 No	5 Yes

DEPRESSION

1	1 No	2 No	3 No	4 Yes	5 Yes
2	1 Yes	2 Yes	3 Yes	4 No	5 Yes
3	1 Yes	2 No	3 No	4 No	5 Yes
4	1 No	2 No	3 Yes	4 No	5 Yes

INSOMNIA and ANXIETY

1	1 Yes	2 No	3 Yes	4 Yes	5 No
2	1 Yes	2 Yes	3 Yes	4 Yes	5 Yes

3	1 Yes	2 Yes	3 No	4 Yes	5 No
4	1 No	2 Yes	3 Yes	4 No	5 Yes

THROMBO-EMBOLISM and HEREDITARY HAEMORRHAGIC DISORDERS

1	1 Yes	2 No	3 Yes	4 Yes	5 No
2	1 Yes	2 Yes	3 No	4 Yes	5 Yes
3	1 Yes	2 Yes	3 No	4 Yes	5 No
4	1 No	2 Yes	3 Yes	4 No	5 Yes
5	1 No	2 No	3 Yes	4 No	5 Yes
6	1 Yes	2 No	3 No	4 No	5 Yes

MALIGNANT DISEASE

1	1 Yes	2 No	3 Yes	4 Yes	5 No
2	1 Yes	2 No	3 No	4 Yes	5 No
3	1 No	2 Yes	3 Yes	4 No	5 Yes
4	1 No	2 Yes	3 Yes	4 Yes	5 No
5	1 Yes	2 Yes	3 Yes	4 No	5 Yes

EPILEPSY

1	1 Yes	2 No	3 Yes	4 Yes	5 No
2	1 No	2 Yes	3 Yes	4 Yes	5 Yes
3	1 Yes	2 Yes	3 No	4 Yes	5 Yes

VITAMIN DEFICIENCY STATE

1	1 Yes	2 No	3 No	4 No	5 Yes
2	1 Yes	2 Yes	3 No	4 Yes	5 No
3	1 Yes	2 Yes	3 No	4 No	5 Yes

MEDICAL EMERGENCIES

1	1 Yes	2 Yes	3 Yes	4 No	5 Yes
2	1 Yes	2 No	3 Yes	4 Yes	5 Yes
3	1 No	2 No	3 Yes	4 Yes	5 Yes
4	1 Yes	2 Yes	3 Yes	4 No	5 No
5	1 No	2 Yes	3 No	4 Yes	5 Yes

FLUORIDES and FLUORIDATION

1	1 No	2 No	3 Yes	4 Yes	5 Yes
2	1 Yes	2 Yes	3 Yes	4 Yes	5 No
3	1 Yes	2 Yes	3 Yes	4 Yes	5 No

INDEX

local 53-62 *see also* Local anaesthesia
machines 41-2
recovery from 37-8
stages 38-9
Anaesthetics
general, mode of action 35-9
during pregnancy 26
Analeptics 90
Analgesics, during pregnancy 26
Anaphylaxis, drug-induced 194-5
Angina 67-70
β-adrenoceptor blocking drugs
69-70
anxiolytic drugs 70
general features 68
nitrites and nitrates 68-9
oxygen 70
Aniline derivatives in pain 143-5
Antagonists, definition 1
Anthranilic acid derivatives in
inflammation 155-6
Antibiotics
antifungal 125
in chronic obstructive airways
disease 87
prophylaxis 112
against infective endocarditis
117-18
at risk groups 118
see also specific names
Anti-cholinergic drugs
in diarrhoea 106
in peptic ulcer 104
in vomiting 105
Anticoagulants
antagonists 174-5
and dental extractions 203
laboratory control 175
in thrombosis 173-4
Anticonvulsants during pregnancy 26
Antidepressant drugs 162-5
Antifungal antibiotics 125
Antihaemophilic globulin 176-7
Antihistamines
as anti-inflammatory agents 161
in asthma 84
in vomiting 105
Antimicrobial drugs
ideal 108
mode of action 109
prescribing during pregnancy 24
resistance 109
Antiprotozoal drugs 126
Antiviral drugs 126
Anxiety

drug treatment 166-71
application 167-8
classification 166
sleep patterns 166-7
Anxiolytic drugs in angina 70
Aphthous ulcers 101
Ascorbic acid deficiency 192
Asparaginase in malignancy 181
Aspirin
in pain 143
during pregnancy 26
see also Salicylates
Asthma, acute 197-8
drugs 84-6
management 198
presentation 197
Atropine in dysrhythmias 95

Barbiturates
in insomnia and anxiety 170-71
Beclomethasone in asthma 85
Benzodiazepines in anxiety and insomnia
168-9
Benzylpenicillin in infection 113-14,
118
Beri-beri 191
Betamethasone
as anti-inflammatory agent 159-60
prescribing during pregnancy 24
properties 7
Bethanidine in hypertension 74
Biguanide drugs 139
Binding
of anaesthetics to protein 36
of drugs 10
Bisacodyl in constipation 103, 107
Blood
disorders and oral ulceration 99
see also Haemorrhagic diseases
loss in anaemia 65
pressure in hypertension 71-2
British National Formulary 27
Bronchodilators in chronic obstructive
airways disease 87

Carbamazepine in epilepsy 189
Carbenicillin sodium in infection 116
Carbenoxolone sodium in peptic
102, 104
Carbocaine *see* Mepivacaine